YOUNGER AND HEALTHIER FOR LIFE

The New Science of Autojuvenation Can Help You Feel Fantastic and Look Your Best.

JOE C. ZIRKLE

TABLE OF CONTENTS

INTRODUCTION

Do you experience sadness, food preoccupation, mood fluctuations, or focus issues? You are significantly more in control of your ideas, feelings, and conduct than you may think, regardless of the situation. In Change Your Diet, Change Your Mind, Dr. Georgia Ede demonstrates that, although pharmaceuticals may provide some comfort, food is the most effective means of altering brain chemistry because it is the primary source of brain chemicals.

In this thought-provoking and enlightening manual, Dr. Ede shows us why almost everything we believe to be true regarding foods that support brain health is false. We've been led to believe that superfoods, supplements, and plant-based diets high in whole grains and legumes are the best ways to safeguard our brains, but the data shows that these methods not only frequently fail, but some may even be detrimental to our brain health.

The truth about brain food is that antioxidants are not the solution, vegan diets are not healthier, and meat is not harmful.

You will be able to: change your mind; change your diet.

Recognize how erratic nutrition headlines and nonsensical dietary recommendations are influenced by flawed study techniques.

Consider the advantages and disadvantages of your favorite foods so that you may make an educated decision about what to eat.

Check for symptoms of insulin resistance, a metabolic disorder that goes undiagnosed yet deprives your brain of the energy it needs to function.

Choose from a variety of ketogenic and moderate-carb diets to suit your dietary needs and desired level of fitness to enhance your mental well-being.

Dr. Ede will pique your interest in the wonderful world of food and its function in nourishing, protecting, and energizing your brain by drawing on a wide range of scientific disciplines, including biochemistry, neuroscience, and botany.

First Chapter

What are the causes of aging?

The decline of physiological capabilities required for survival and reproduction over time is known as aging. It is important to distinguish between senescence-related disorders like cancer and heart disease, which impact individuals, and the phenotypic changes associated with senescence, which affect all members of the species.

Entropy is the ultimate winner. There is a limited amount of time that each multicellular creature may develop and preserve its identity utilizing solar energy. The organism then ages as degradation takes precedence over production. The time-related decline of physiological processes required for reproduction and survival is known as aging. All members of a species are impacted by the traits of aging, as opposed to aging-related disorders like cancer and heart disease.

Aging is not something that many evolutionary biologists would argue is a part of an animal's genetic repertoire. Instead, they would view aging as the animal's natural state, which happens when it satisfies the conditions of natural selection. Once the young have been born and reared, the animal may pass away. Indeed, this is precisely what occurs in a wide variety of creatures, including salmon and moths. The adults perish as soon as the eggs are fertilized and laid. Recent research, however, suggests that senescence has genetic components and that modifying genes or food might affect a species' genetically defined life span feature.

Maximum Life Expectancy and Life Span

One trait of the species is its maximum life span. That represents the longest a member of that species has been known to live. It is estimated that the greatest human lifespan is 121 years. Although the lifespans of lake trout and tortoises are uncertain, they are both thought to exceed 150 years. A laboratory mouse has a maximum life span of 4.5 years, while a domestic dog has an approximate 20-year lifespan.

A Drosophila fruit fly can live up to three months if it makes it to eclosion (in the wild, approximately 90% of them die as larvae).

But one cannot expect to live to be 121 years old, and the majority of wild mice do not survive to see their first birthday. Life expectancy, or how long a member of a species can expect to live, is a population trait rather than a trait of a species. The age at which half of the population still exists is the standard definition. In the 1780s, a newborn born in England may have anticipated living to be 35 years old. At that same time, the average life expectancy in Massachusetts was 28 years. For the majority of human history, this was the typical range of life expectancy. In several parts of the world (Afghanistan, Togo, Cambodia, and several more nations), the life expectancy is still less than 40 years. In the US, a kid born in 1986 can anticipate living for 71 years for a man and 78 years for a woman.

Our awareness of human aging is rather new, since most times and places humans did not live much past 40 years of age. In colonial America, 65-year-olds were uncommon, but they are now a common sight.

Figure 18.35 shows some plots of survival curves for female Homo sapiens in the United States. By the age of 58, half of American women had died in 1900. By the age of 81, half of American women had died in 1980. Senescence and age-related illnesses are therefore far more prevalent now than they were a century ago. Around 1900, people did not have the "luxury" of passing away from cancer or heart attacks. People over 50 are typically affected by these disorders. Instead, infectious diseases and parasites were the cause of death—and they still are in many parts of the world—for human beings (Arking 1998). The more common human sense phenotype, which includes graying hair, sagging and wrinkled skin, joint stiffness, osteoporosis (loss of bone calcium), loss of muscle fibers and muscular strength, memory loss, deteriorating eyesight, and a slowing of sexual responsiveness, was also uncommon until recently. Shakespeare wrote, "Sans teeth, sans eyes, sans taste, sans everything," about individuals who did not succumb to senescence in As You Like It.

Reasons for Getting Older

Every species exhibits a distinct senescent phenotype. However, what triggers it? There are various ways to ask this question. The cellular level of organization will be our main focus. There is evidence supporting a wide range of views even in this case, and the reason for aging is still up for debate.

Oxidative harm

According to a popular view, aging is caused by changes in our metabolism. This idea states that aging is a natural byproduct of metabolism and doesn't require mutations. Reactive oxygen species (ROS) are produced when the mitochondria fail to adequately degrade 2–3% of the oxygen atoms that are taken in by them. The superoxide ion, the hydroxyl radical, and hydrogen peroxide are some of these ROS. Proteins, nucleic acids, and cell membranes can all be oxidized and harmed by ROS. The finding that Drosophila that overexpress enzymes that break down reactive oxygen species (ROS)—catalase, which breaks down peroxide, and superoxide dismutase—live 30–40% longer than controls lends credence to this notion.

Furthermore, flies with mutations in the methuselah gene—named for the 969-year-old man in the Bible—live 35% longer than flies of the wild type. According to Lin et al. (1998), the methusaleh mutants exhibit increased resistance to paraquat, a toxin that acts by producing ROS inside cells. These results provide evidence for the involvement of ROS in the aging process, in addition to suggesting that aging is controlled by genetics. In addition, elegans individuals with mutations that boost the production of ROS-degrading enzymes have considerably longer lifespans than worms of the wild type.

It's not as evident how ROS contribute to mammalian aging. Premature aging is not caused by mutations in mice that render several ROS-degrading enzymes inactive (Ho et al., 1997; Melov et al., 1998). Mammals, as opposed to invertebrates, might have more genetic redundancy, and other genes might be activated to create related ROS-degrading enzymes. A study by Migliaccio et al. (1999) found that mutant mice survive one-third longer than their littermates of the wild type. These mice are deficient in p66shc, a specific protein.

The absence of p66shc appears to provide them with greater cellular resistance to ROS, which in turn protects proteins and membranes from oxygen-induced stress throughout normal development. The p66shc protein may have a role in modulating animal life lengths and be a part of a signal transduction pathway that triggers apoptosis in response to oxygen exposure.

Another piece of evidence that suggests ROS may have a role in mammalian aging is the ability of caloric restriction to slow down mammalian aging. It's unclear, though, if caloric restriction prevents ROS generation or if it has any additional impacts. Furthermore, both vitamins E and C decrease reactive oxygen species (ROS), and adding vitamin E to food lengthens the life span of nematodes and flies. Nevertheless, it is more difficult to interpret the data in mammals, and there is insufficient proof that ROS inhibitors are equally effective in vertebrates.

general deterioration and hereditary instability

One of the earliest ideas of aging to explain the overall scenescent phenotype is the "wear-and-tear" theory.

Little traumas to the body accumulate with age. Our genes encode enzymes with decreasing efficiency as the number of point mutations rises. Furthermore, the cell would produce a high proportion of defective proteins if a mutation happened in any one component of the machinery that synthesizes proteins (Orgel 1963). The rate of mutations should rise dramatically if the enzymes that synthesize DNA undergo mutations; Murray and Holliday (1981) have reported on defective DNA polymerases in senescent cells. Similarly, DNA repair may play a role in delaying senescence, and organisms with higher levels of DNA repair enzymes in their cells have longer lifespans. Furthermore, human premature aging diseases can result from genetic flaws in DNA repair enzymes.

Harm to the mitochondrial genome

According to Johnson et al. (1999), the rate of mutation in mitochondria is 10–20 times higher than the rate of mutation in nuclear DNA. It is believed that mutations in the mitochondria may (1) cause errors in the synthesis of energy, (2) cause defective electron transport to produce ROS, and/or (3) cause apoptosis.

Numerous animals, including humans, exhibit age-dependent reductions in mitochondrial function (Boffoli et al., 1994). According to a recent study (Michikawa et al. 1999), the mitochondrial genome contains "hot spots" for age-related mutations, and the replication frequency of these mutant mitochondria is higher than that of wild-type mitochondria. As a result, the mutant mitochondria are able to outcompete the wild-type mitochondria and ultimately take control of the cell and its offspring. Furthermore, the alterations might increase the production of ROS as well as increase the vulnerability of mitochondrial DNA to damage from ROS.

Reduction in telomere length

At the ends of chromosomes are repetitive DNA sequences called telomeres. They are not maintained by telomerase, and DNA polymerase cannot duplicate them. They will also get shorter with every cell division. With every cell division, telomerase appends the telomere to the chromosome. Since telomerase is absent from the majority of mammalian somatic tissues, it has been suggested

(Salk 1982; Harley et al. 1990) that telomere shortening may function as a "clock" that finally stops cells from proliferating. Human fibroblasts have a limited capacity for division and shortening telomeres when cultivated. These cells can divide indefinitely if they are engineered to produce telomerase (Bodnar et al., 1998; Vaziri and Benchimol, 1998).

But since humans have significantly shorter telomeres than mice, there is no relationship between telomere length and life expectancy, nor is there a relationship between telomere length and age in humans (Cristofalo et al. 1998). If telomerase were the primary determinant of the rate of aging, telomerase-deficient animals would not exhibit severe aging abnormalities (Rudolph et al., 1999). Some have proposed that telomere-dependent suppression of cell division functions more as a preventive measure against cancer than as an "aging clock."

Programs for genetic aging

Aging has been linked to multiple genes. Hutchinson-Gilford progeria syndrome in humans results in children who age quickly and pass away at a young age of 12 (typically from heart failure). Its symptoms include arteriosclerosis, resorbed bone mass, hair loss, and thin skin with age spots. It is brought on by a dominant mutant gene. In mice, mutations in the klotho gene result in a condition that is comparable (Kuro-o et al., 1997). Although the roles of the products of these genes are unknown, it is believed that they have a role in squelching aging phenotypes. The time of senescence may be greatly influenced by these proteins.

In C. elegans, aging appears to be influenced by at least two different genetic mechanisms. Making the choice to either continue growing or stay a larva is the first pathway. Following its hatch, the C. The larva of C. elegans goes through four instar stages before becoming an adult or, in the event of overcrowding or a lack of food, entering a nonfeeding, metabolically inactive dauer stage. Rather than developing into an adult that only lives a few weeks, it can continue to exist as a dauer larva for up to six months. It will live for the same amount of time after emerging from the dauer stage as if it had never been a dauer larva.

During the dauer stage, further defenses against ROS are synthesized, and adult development is blocked. Adult development is permitted if a few of the genes in this pathway are disrupted, but the ROS defense mechanisms are still in place. Adults of this kind survive two to four times longer than adults of the wild type (Figure 18.38; Friedman and Johnson 1988). The gonads are involved in the second route. The somatic cells of the gonads function to extend the nematode's life, while germ cells seem to limit it.

Despite advances in disease prevention and treatment, which have extended human life expectancy, we are nevertheless plagued by the general aging phenomenon that is unique to our species. If we don't address the general aging problem, we run the risk of becoming like the Greek mythological character Tithonios, who was granted endless life but not eternal youth by the gods.

Types, Causes, and Prevention of Aging

Although we all experience aging, relatively little is known about it.

Although it's easy to enumerate all the negative effects of aging, such as memory loss, wrinkles, and the loss of lean muscle mass, nobody truly knows what aging is, why it occurs, or if it can be stopped.

Section Two

Aging Types

When we go deeper into the aging process, we find that there are a number of hypotheses that explain why and how our bodies age in different ways.

Aging Cells

Before the genetic material can no longer be reliably replicated, a cell can reproduce itself roughly 50 times. Cellular senescence is the term used to describe this failure of replication, in which the cell loses its functional properties. The hallmark of cellular aging, which corresponds to biological aging, is the build-up of senescent cells.

Cellular senescence progresses more quickly the more damage that free radicals and environmental variables inflict on cells, necessitating increased cell replication.

Ageing Hormonally

Hormones have a major impact on aging, particularly in childhood, when they aid in the formation of secondary male or female traits and help grow bones and muscles.

Many hormones will eventually start to produce less of an effect, which will cause changes in the skin (such as wrinkles and elasticity loss) as well as a decrease in bone density, sex desire, and muscular tone.

Total Injury

The external forces that can accumulate over time are what lead to aging caused by accumulative damage, often known as "wear and tear." Toxin exposure, UV radiation, eating unhealthily, and pollution are just a few of the things that might harm the body. 4

These outside elements have the potential to gradually harm cells' DNA directly (partially by subjecting them to severe or ongoing inflammation). The body's capacity to heal itself may be compromised by the cumulative injury, hastening the aging process.

Ageing Metabolically

Your cells are continuously converting food into energy as you go about your daily activities. This process creates byproducts, some of which may be detrimental to your health. Although necessary, the metabolization process can gradually harm cells; this is known as metabolic aging.

The Process of Aging

In spite of our age-obsessed culture's obsession with "slowing down aging" and extending life, the fundamental reality of aging is inevitable. Whatever you do, there will be some significant changes to your physique.

For instance, the muscles around the rib cage will start to weaken, lung tissues will start to lose their flexibility, and a person's overall lung function will start to decline by the time they turn 20.

In a similar vein, as we age, our body's ability to absorb nutrients and process certain foods will be compromised by a slowdown in the creation of digestive enzymes.

Ways to Reduce the Signs of Aging

It is impossible to stop aging. Having said that, there are a number of actions you can take to lessen the impact of environmental influences on aging:

Consume healthfully. Saturated fat, added sugar, and salt cause havoc in the body and raise the risk of heart disease, diabetes, and hypertension. Increase your consumption of fruits, vegetables, whole grains, low-fat dairy, lean meat, and fish to prevent these aging-related issues.

Examine the labels. If you purchase packaged goods for convenience, make sure to read the labels and follow the guidelines to keep your daily intake of sugar to about 25 mg, saturated fat to less than 10% of calories, and sodium to less than 1,500 mg.

Give up smoking. Giving up cigarettes lowers your risk of cancer and increases blood pressure and circulation. There are effective cessation tools that can assist, even if it often takes numerous efforts to finally break the habit.

Work out.

The majority of adults do not get the recommended amount of exercise (5 days a week, 30 minutes of moderate to intense activity) for optimal health. Nevertheless, compared to not exercising at all, 15 minutes a day of moderate activity can increase longevity. 10

Make friends. Socialization influences our psychological engagement and may also have an impact on our longevity. 11 Keep up positive, healthy interactions with other people. Maintain relationships with the people you care about, and actively seek out new acquaintances.

Get enough rest. Chronic sleep deprivation has been associated with worse health and shorter life spans. 12 You may prolong your life and feel better by practicing good sleep hygiene and obtaining 7 to 8 hours of sleep every night.

Lessen your tension. Prolonged anxiety and stress can be harmful to your body because they cause the inflammatory stress hormone cortisol to be released. The indirect inflammatory load on cells may be reduced by mastering mind-body therapies and relaxation strategies for stress management.

The telltale indications of aging start to show at some point in life, usually in the thirtys. They are present in all bodily systems, including our skin, bones, joints, neurological, digestive, and cardiovascular systems, as well as our vital indicators (such as blood pressure). Early in life, certain aging changes can occur. For instance, starting around the age of 20, your metabolism begins to progressively decrease. On the other hand, hearing changes typically don't start until after the age of 50.

We still don't fully comprehend the intricate web of interactions that leads to our aging process. We are aware that aging is influenced by a wide range of factors, including heredity, nutrition, exercise, disease, and a lot of other things.

Since the 1990s, a number of outstanding biological research studies have revealed genes that have a significant impact on how quickly cells and animals age. The good news from this research is that longer-living organisms appear to have more vitality as well; over the majority of their extended lives, longer-living animals maintain relatively decent health.

While none of these findings comes close to offering a "fountain of youth" for people, some scientists predict that advances in our understanding of aging in the twenty-first century will result in the creation of medications that can both prolong human life and enhance human health. Naturally, if that occurs, everything will only work out well if there is enough space, employment, and other resources available for everyone who is added.

Here are some illustrations of how some of our main body systems are impacted by aging.

Tissues, organs, and cells:

The ability of cells to divide declines.

Every cell has telomeres, which are the endpoints of its chromosomes. Over time, these ends gradually shorten until the cell dies.

Waste materials build up.

The intercellular connective tissue stiffens.

Many organs' maximal functional capability declines.

Blood vessels and the heart:

The cardiac wall becomes thicker.

Less efficient heart muscle requires more effort to pump the same volume of blood.

The body's principal artery, the aorta, gets less flexible, stiffer, and thicker.

Atherosclerosis steadily develops in many of the body's arteries, including those that carry blood to the heart and brain; however, some people never have significant symptoms from the illness.

Vital indicators:

The body finds it more difficult to regulate its temperature.

After exercise, the heart rate takes longer to return to normal.

Muscles, joints, and bones:

Bones weaken and thin over time.

Joints lose their flexibility and stiffness.

Joint bone and cartilage begin to deteriorate.

Muscle mass decreases in bulk and strength.

Digestive system:

Food passes through the digestive system more slowly.

The production of digestive fluids is reduced in the stomach, liver, pancreas, and small intestine.

Nervous system and brain:

The brain and spinal cord's neural cell count declines.

Neural cell connections become fewer in number.

In the brain, abnormal formations called plaques and tangles can occur.

Hearing and seeing:

The iris stiffens, and the retinas become thinner.

The clarity of the lenses decreases.

The ear canal's walls get thinner.

The auditory drums thicken.

Nails, hair, and skin:

Skin thins and loses its elasticity.

Sweat gland production is reduced.

Slower nail growth

Graying hair and non-growth in certain areas

Signs of aging

Although we all age differently and to varying degrees, there are some common aging impacts that we all encounter. The following are a few typical aging signs and symptoms:

Heightened vulnerability to infection.

Increased chance of hypothermia or heat stroke

Modest drop in height when our spines' bones deteriorate and become shorter

More easily broken bones

Alterations in the joints, from mild stiffness to severe arthritis.

Bent-over position

Reduced and sluggish motion

Reduction in total energy

Constipation

Incontinence in the urine

Modest cognitive, memory, and reasoning slowdown (delirium, dementia, and severe memory loss, on the other hand, are not typical aspects of aging).

Diminished reflexes, impaired balance, and poor coordination

decline in sharpness of vision

reduced vision in the periphery

a certain amount of hearing loss.

Drooping and wrinkled skin

Graying or whitening of the hair

Loss of muscular tissue contributes to weight loss, which occurs after age 65 for women and after age 55 for men.

Identifying aging

Not all of the natural changes that occur to the body and mind as we age are normal. There are a lot of false beliefs regarding what aspects of aging are typical. For example, unlike what many people think, senility is not a normal side effect of aging.

It's critical that you discuss any changes you notice with your doctor. You can learn to distinguish between signs of normal aging and those that are not from your doctor. Your doctor might recommend you to a specialist if needed.

Anticipated longevity of aging

The process of aging is progressive and ongoing, lasting until death.

Keeping oneself from aging

Both the passage of time and our genes are unchangeable. We may, however, lower our risk for a number of illnesses and ailments that grow more common as we age by making lifestyle adjustments. Immunizations and screening tests are other ways that we can prevent illness. testing for screening. Screening tests have the ability to identify diseases in their early, perhaps curable, stages. But as you age, the possible advantages of screening exams and procedures decrease. It is true that screening tests may not always be beneficial. For example, extra, riskier, and needless testing might be ordered if the test is mistakenly positive, meaning it suggests that a person may have a condition even though he doesn't.

Consult your physician to ascertain whether a certain screening test is appropriate for you. For instance, if your chance of contracting a certain disease is extremely low to begin with, you might not need to get screened for it.

It might not be worth taking the test in the first place if you know you would not accept treatment for a certain condition if it was found by a screening exam. Alternatively, there would be little point in doing a screening test for an illness if finding and treating it did not improve or prolong your life. The decision on whether screening tests are beneficial rests solely with you and your healthcare provider.

Vaccinations. Adults are most frequently advised to get the following vaccinations:

Influenza, annually

pneumococcal pneumonia vaccination for individuals 65 years of age and older, as well as those between the ages of 19 and 64 who are susceptible to pneumococcal infection (due to conditions like lung or chronic heart disease).

One injection each of tetanus, diphtheria, and pertussis, followed every ten years by tetanus and diphtheria.

Shingles vaccination against herpes zoster for individuals 50 years of age and older, regardless of prior shingles episodes.

Meningococcal vaccination if your doctor advises you are particularly susceptible to this illness.

Vaccination against the human papillomavirus, based on your age and risk profile.

Vaccinations against the hepatitis A and B viruses, if you were not given them as a kid and if you are at a higher risk of contracting this infection.

These are broad suggestions for senior citizens. It might be advisable for some older people to receive additional vaccinations. Certain vaccinations that are normally advised against should not be administered to others, such as those with compromised immune systems. Consult your physician to sort all of this out.

Taking care of aging

It is crucial to consider not just how long you will live but also how well you will live as you get older. As you get older, the following tactics can help you preserve and possibly even improve your quality of life.

Avoid smoking. In addition to raising the risk of numerous cancers, smoking also raises the risk of heart disease, osteoporosis, and stroke.

It even seems that smoking deteriorates memory. The good news is that years of smoking can cause harm that can be partially or completely undone by quitting.

Include mental and physical activity in your daily routine. Exercise benefits both the body and the mind. Exercise keeps your bones and heart healthy, as well as your weight under control. Exercise can also include non-exercise activities like housework or gardening. Additionally, research indicates that individuals who engage in physical activity have a decreased risk of dementia and are more likely to maintain mental activity. Additionally, maintaining mental activity prevents memory loss.

Consume a diet high in fruits, vegetables, and whole grains, and replace bad saturated fats with monounsaturated and polyunsaturated fats. A diet like this shields you from numerous illnesses, such as the three leading causes of death: heart disease, cancer, and stroke.

Keep your weight and body type in a healthy range. Our metabolism slows down as we age, making it more difficult to burn calories.

However, being overweight can raise your chance of developing diabetes, heart disease, stroke, and several types of cancer. Additionally crucial is body shape. The risk of heart attack and stroke is higher in men and women who carry excess weight around their abdomens than it is in those who carry it around their hips.

Test your thinking. Reading, crossword puzzle solving, learning to play an instrument, and even having stimulating conversations have all been shown to help maintain mental acuity.

Create a robust social network. Maintaining strong and fulfilling relationships with family and friends as you age is crucial, as is making new ones when you can. According to certain research, having social connections may help prevent dementia and maintain mental acuity. Strong social ties may extend your life, according to other research.

To safeguard your hearing, vision, and overall well-being, adhere to preventative care recommendations.

Brush, floss, and visit the dentist frequently.

Numerous negative effects of poor dental health may include inadequate nourishment, needless discomfort, and maybe an increased risk of heart disease and stroke.

Talk to your doctor about whether you require any medicine to help you maintain your health, such as to treat osteoporosis, decrease cholesterol, or control high blood pressure.

Aging: What is it?

Aging gracefully is evident in many ways, such as wrinkles, gray hair, a slightly hunched posture, and occasional "senior moments" of forgetfulness. However, why do those things occur? Aging: What is it?

Thirteen trillion cells make up each of us. Each of our tissues and organs is made up of numerous natural components that the cells have created to hold each other together.

Every cell in our body, including our tissues and organs, starts to age as soon as we are conceived.

Naturally, in the early stages of life, we continue to grow and divide into new cells. The body is growing and expanding, but we are not able to see the small aging of the cells.

The telltale indications of aging start to show at some point in life, usually in the thirtys. They are present in all bodily systems, including our skin, bones, joints, neurological, digestive, and cardiovascular systems, as well as our vital indicators (such as blood pressure). Early in life, certain aging changes can occur. For instance, starting around the age of 20, your metabolism begins to progressively decrease. On the other hand, hearing changes typically don't start until after the age of 50.

We still don't fully comprehend the intricate web of interactions that leads to our aging process. We are aware that aging is influenced by a wide range of factors, including heredity, nutrition, exercise, disease, and a lot of other things.

Since the 1990s, a number of outstanding biological research studies have revealed genes that have a significant impact on how quickly cells and animals age.

The good news from this research is that longer-living organisms appear to have more vitality as well; over the majority of their extended lives, longer-living animals maintain relatively decent health.

While none of these findings comes close to offering a "fountain of youth" for people, some scientists predict that advances in our understanding of aging in the twenty-first century will result in the creation of medications that can both prolong human life and enhance human health. Naturally, if that occurs, everything will only work out well if there is enough space, employment, and other resources available for everyone who is added.

Here are some illustrations of how some of our main body systems are impacted by aging.

Tissues, organs, and cells:

The ability of cells to divide declines.

Every cell has telomeres, which are the endpoints of its chromosomes. Over time, these ends gradually shorten until the cell dies.

Waste materials build up.

The intercellular connective tissue stiffens.

Many organs' maximal functional capability declines.

Blood vessels and the heart:

The cardiac wall becomes thicker.

Less efficient heart muscle requires more effort to pump the same volume of blood.

The body's principal artery, the aorta, gets less flexible, stiffer, and thicker.

Atherosclerosis steadily develops in many of the body's arteries, including those that carry blood to the heart and brain; however, some people never have significant symptoms from the illness.

vital indicators:

The body finds it more difficult to regulate its temperature.

After exercise, the heart rate takes longer to return to normal.

Muscles, joints, and bones:

Bones weaken and thin over time.

Joints lose their flexibility and stiffness.

Joint bone and cartilage begin to deteriorate.

Muscle mass decreases in bulk and strength.

Digestive system more details:

Food passes through the digestive system more slowly.

The production of digestive fluids is reduced in the stomach, liver, pancreas, and small intestine.

Nervous system and brain:

The brain and spinal cord's neural cell count declines.

Neural cell connections become fewer in number.

In the brain, abnormal formations called plaques and tangles can occur.

Hearing and seeing:

The iris stiffens, and the retinas become thinner.

The clarity of the lenses decreases.

The ear canal's walls get thinner.

The auditory drums thicken.

Nails, hair, and skin:

Skin thins and loses its elasticity.

Sweat gland production is reduced.

Slower nail growth.

Incontinence in the urine

Modest cognitive, memory, and reasoning slowdown (delirium, dementia, and severe memory loss, on the other hand, are not typical aspects of aging).

Diminished reflexes, impaired balance, and poor coordination

Decline in sharpness of vision

Reduced vision in the periphery

A certain amount of hearing loss.

Drooping and wrinkled skin

Graying or whitening of the hair

Loss of muscular tissue contributes to weight loss, which occurs after age 65 for women and after age 55 for men.

Identifying aging

Not all of the natural changes that occur to the body and mind as we age are normal. There are a lot of false beliefs regarding what aspects of aging are typical. For example, unlike what many people think, senility is not a normal side effect of aging.

It's critical that you discuss any changes you notice with your doctor. You can learn to distinguish between signs of normal aging and those that are not from your doctor. Your doctor might recommend you to a specialist if needed.

Anticipated longevity of aging

The process of aging is progressive and ongoing, lasting until death.

Keeping oneself from aging

Both the passage of time and our genes are unchangeable. We may, however, lower our risk for a number of illnesses and ailments that grow more common as we age by making lifestyle adjustments. Immunizations and screening tests are other ways that we can prevent illness. testing for screening. Screening tests have the ability to identify diseases in their early, perhaps curable, stages. But as you age, the possible advantages of screening exams and procedures decrease. It is true that screening tests may not always be beneficial. For example, extra, riskier, and needless testing might be ordered if the test is mistakenly positive, meaning it suggests that a person may have a condition even though he doesn't.

Consult your physician to ascertain whether a certain screening test is appropriate for you. For instance, if your chance of contracting a certain disease is extremely low to begin with, you might not need to get screened for it. It might not be worth taking the test in the first place if you know you would not accept treatment for a certain condition if it was found by a screening exam. Alternatively, there would be little point in doing a screening test for an illness if finding and treating it did not improve or prolong your life. The decision on whether screening tests are beneficial rests solely with you and your healthcare provider.

Vaccinations. Adults are most frequently advised to get the following vaccinations:

Influenza, annually

pneumococcal pneumonia vaccination for individuals 65 years of age and older, as well as those between the ages of 19 and 64 who are susceptible to pneumococcal infection (due to conditions like lung or chronic heart disease).

One injection each of tetanus, diphtheria, and pertussis, followed every ten years by tetanus and diphtheria.

Shingles vaccination against herpes zoster for individuals 50 years of age and older, regardless of prior shingles episodes

Meningococcal vaccination if your doctor advises you are particularly susceptible to this illness.

Vaccination against the human papillomavirus, based on your age and risk profile.

Vaccinations against the hepatitis A and B viruses, if you were not given them as a kid and if you are at a higher risk of contracting this infection.

These are broad suggestions for senior citizens. It might be advisable for some older people to receive additional vaccinations. Certain vaccinations that are normally advised against should not be administered to others, such as those with compromised immune systems. Consult your physician to sort all of this out.

Taking care of aging

It is crucial to consider not just how long you will live but also how well you will live as you get older. As you get older, the following tactics can help you preserve and possibly even improve your quality of life.

Avoid smoking. In addition to raising the risk of numerous cancers, smoking also raises the risk of heart disease, osteoporosis, and stroke. It even seems that smoking deteriorates memory. The good news is that years of smoking can cause harm that can be partially or completely undone by quitting.

Include mental and physical activity in your daily routine. Exercise benefits both the body and the mind. Exercise keeps your bones and heart healthy, as well as your weight under control. Exercise can also include non-exercise activities like housework or gardening. Additionally, research indicates that individuals who engage in physical activity have a decreased risk of dementia and are more likely to maintain mental activity. Additionally, maintaining mental activity prevents memory loss.

Consume a diet high in fruits, vegetables, and whole grains, and replace bad saturated fats with monounsaturated and polyunsaturated fats. A diet like this shields you from numerous illnesses, such as the three leading causes of death: heart disease, cancer, and stroke.

Keep your weight and body type in a healthy range. Our metabolism slows down as we age, making it more difficult to burn calories. However, being overweight can raise your chance of developing diabetes, heart disease, stroke, and several types of cancer. Additionally crucial is body shape. The risk of heart attack and stroke is higher in men and women who carry excess weight around their abdomens than it is in those who carry it around their hips.

Test your thinking. Reading, crossword puzzle solving, learning to play an instrument, and even having stimulating conversations have all been shown to help maintain mental acuity.

Create a robust social network. Maintaining strong and fulfilling relationships with family and friends as you age is crucial, as is making new ones when you can.

According to certain research, having social connections may help prevent dementia and maintain mental acuity. Strong social ties may extend your life, according to other research.

To safeguard your hearing, vision, and overall well-being, adhere to preventative care recommendations.

Brush, floss, and visit the dentist frequently. Numerous negative effects of poor dental health may include inadequate nourishment, needless discomfort, and maybe an increased risk of heart disease and stroke.

Talk to your doctor about whether you require any medicine to help you maintain your health, such as to treat osteoporosis, decrease cholesterol, or control high blood pressure.

When to contact a specialist

If you observe any changes that defy what is expected with aging, give your doctor a call. For instance, while a slight slowdown in thinking and occasional forgetfulness are natural, delirium, dementia, and severe memory loss are not signs of aging and should be discussed with your physician.

Forecast Even though aging is inevitable, there are things you can do to lower your chance of illness and keep your quality of life intact as you age.

Theories about genetics

According to one hypothesis of aging, an organism's or cell's life span is genetically predetermined; an animal's genes carry a "programme" that establishes its lifespan, much like genetics determines eye color. The likelihood of lengthy life expectancy among parents who have lived long lives lends credence to this notion. Moreover, the life spans of identical twins are longer than those of non-twin siblings.

Telomeres, which are repeating sections of DNA (deoxyribonucleic acid) found at the ends of chromosomes, are central to the genetic hypothesis of aging. Since several repeats are lost with each cell division, the maximum life span of a cell is determined by the number of repeats in its telomere. The cell reaches a crisis point when its telomeres are too short to allow it to divide any further. Consequently, the cell perishes.

Telomeres are susceptible to genetic factors that change an organism's pace of aging, according to research. Reduced telomere length and a faster rate of biological aging have been linked to mutations in the TERC gene (telomerase RNA [ribonucleic acid] component), which encodes an RNA segment of the telomerase enzyme, in humans. The normal purpose of telomerase is to stop telomeres from getting too short; however, TERC mutations cause the enzyme to behave differently. Additionally, it seems that TERC affects an individual's telomere length from birth. When comparing TERC variant carriers to noncarriers of the same chronological age, it is thought that carriers are physiologically several years older. The acceleration of biological aging is probably partly caused by environmental variables like obesity and smoking, which raise a carrier's risk of developing age-related disorders very early in adulthood.

Another genetic explanation of aging, which holds that "errors" in the synthesis of essential proteins, including enzymes, cause cell death, is supported by mutations of genes affecting telomere length.

A molecule of the enzyme that does not "work" properly could be the result of minute variations in the information transmitted from chromosomal DNA molecules to RNA molecules (the "messenger" material) to the correct assembly of the huge and complex enzyme molecules. This is exactly the outcome that occurs when the TERC gene is mutated. These mutations impair the telomerase enzyme's ability to function normally.

A tiny percentage of cells experience mutations when they proliferate and divide. Then, when the cells divide once more, this alteration in the genetic code is replicated. According to the "somatic mutation" theory of aging, the slow buildup of abnormally functioning mutant cells is what causes aging.

Theories that are not genetic

All of these theories try to explain aging in terms of cellular and molecular changes, but they also concentrate on variables that can affect the expression of a genetically determined "program." In actuality, age differences are considerably more noticeable in an individual's total performance than in measurable cellular processes.

The decline in muscle function with age is significantly larger than any discernible alterations in the enzyme levels of the corresponding muscles. It is plausible that an individual's aging process may be caused by a malfunction in the control systems necessary for sophisticated performance. Another possible cause of aging in cells is the build-up of harmful reactive chemicals that are generated as byproducts of regular cellular processes like respiration. Aging is viewed as a complicated psychosocial process in some nongenetic theories.

Theory of wear and tear

According to the "wear-and-tear" notion, cells and animals just age like machinery does. But unlike machines, animals can heal themselves to some extent, so this idea does not match the realities of a biological system. Assumption number one of the wear-and-tear theory is that waste products build up inside cells and impede their ability to function. Muscle cells in the heart and nerve cells in humans and other animals have been shown to accumulate very insoluble particles called "age pigments."

The theory of cross-linking

Tendons, epidermis, and even blood vessels become less elastic as we age. This is because the fibrous protein called collagen, which gives these tissues their elasticity, forms cross-links inside and between their molecules. According to the "cross-linking" theory of aging, comparable cross-links develop in other molecules that are crucial to biology, like enzymes. These cross-links have the potential to change the form and structure of the enzyme molecules, impairing their ability to function within the cell.

The theory of autoimmunity

According to a different hypothesis of aging, immune responses that are often directed against foreign proteins, tissues, or organisms that cause disease start to target the person's own body cells. Stated differently, the immune system becomes less capable of differentiating between "self" and alien proteins. The "autoimmune" theory of aging is not supported by experimental data but rather by clinical evidence.

Notion

According to the "glycation" idea, glucose mediates the aging process. Throughout life, glycation—the process by which simple sugars, like glucose, attach to components like proteins and lipids—has a significant cumulative impact. These consequences could be comparable to the higher blood glucose levels and shortened life spans seen in those with diabetes.

The theory of oxidative damage

Proteins and other biological components may oxidize as a result of internal reactions in cells. The process of oxidation involves these molecules losing electrons, which makes them unstable and extremely reactive. This ultimately causes the molecules to react with cell components like membranes, causing damage to those components. Any atom or molecule with a single unpaired electron in its outer shell is referred to as a free radical.

The accumulation of oxidative stress and damage with age has led to the development of the free radical hypothesis of aging, which focuses on molecules referred to as reactive oxygen species (ROS).

American gerontologist Denham Harman first put up this notion in the 1950s, and it was partially backed by data showing that aging cells had higher levels of antioxidant proteins, which counteract free radicals and are thought to be a reaction to oxidative stress.

Since mitochondria are the main centers of energy production in the majority of eukaryotic species, the original free radical theory of aging was later expanded to include ROS generated from these organelles (eukaryotic cells are cells with clearly defined nuclei). The premise of the mitochondrial theory of aging was that mitochondria are home to a vicious cycle of oxidative stress whereby mutations in mitochondrial DNA affect the function of proteins involved in the respiration machinery of the organelle, increasing the generation of oxygen radicals that damage DNA. This ultimately leads to the accumulation of mutations in the DNA of the mitochondria and a bioenergetic impairment, which is defined as the mitochondria's inability to generate enough energy for cells to go about their everyday lives.

This ultimately causes tissue dysfunction and degeneration.

According to a related mitochondrial theory of aging, ROS are produced when electrons leaking from the electron transport chain (ETC), which is the main respiration machinery of the organelle, damage ETC proteins and mitochondrial DNA. This damages the mitochondrial DNA and causes additional intracellular ROS levels to rise, ultimately leading to a decline in mitochondrial function.

The molecular-inflammatory theory of aging is another thing to think about. According to this theory, proinflammatory genes are expressed more frequently as a result of age-related oxidative stress activating redox- (oxidation-reduction-) sensitive transcription factors (molecules that regulate gene activity), which results in inflammation in different tissues. This inflammatory cascade gets more pronounced as people age and has been connected to a number of age-related illnesses, including arthritis, cancer, cardiovascular disease, and multiple neurodegenerative diseases.

Chronic inflammation might potentially hasten aging, regardless of the cause—diet, infection, stress, or other variables.

Restricted-calorie mammals mature more slowly and release fewer ROS. Calorie restriction has been linked to these effects because it can reduce the constant state of oxidative stress, delay the accumulation of oxidative damage associated with aging, and improve metabolic efficiency.

One thing that all of the previously suggested theories have in common is that ROS is a major cause of many age-related illnesses.

Theory of psychosociology

A "psychosociological" explanation of aging exists in addition to theories based on molecules and cells. People change with age in terms of behavior, social connections, and activities they participate in. The disengagement, activity, life-course, and continuity theories are the four basic component hypotheses that make up the psychosociological theory of aging. The foundation of disengagement theory is a person's impaired ties with other members of society.

Activity theory highlights the value of continuous social interaction and proposes a connection between an individual's roles and their self-perception. The developmental stages put forth by German-born American psychoanalyst Erik H. Erikson serve as the foundation for life-course theory. Erikson's stages describe maturation as a process that lasts into old age, with new psychosocial demands placed on the individual at each turn. According to continuity theory, despite changes in their health or circumstances, older people attempt to keep and preserve both internal and exterior qualities (such as values, personalities, preferences, and behavioral patterns) throughout their lives.

Section Three

Aging's natural history

Aging and procreation

An organism's life history revolves around its reproductive system, and all other essential processes—such as senescence and death—are molded around it. Understanding the differences between iteroparous and semelparous reproduction is crucial to comprehending biological aging. Single reproductive acts are used by similar creatures to reproduce. Along with many invertebrates and a few vertebrates, like salmon and eels, semelparous plants are annual and biannual. Conversely, iteroparous species reproduce repeatedly across a reproductive duration that typically encompasses a significant portion of their overall life span.

In semparous forms, reproduction occurs close to the end of the organism's life span, followed by a swift senescence that ends in the organism's sudden death.

The senescent phase is typically a crucial component of the reproductive process in plants and is required for its successful completion. For example, the ripening and dropping (abscission) of fruits and the drying of seed pods are integral processes of the overall senescence process that facilitate seed dissemination. Furthermore, hormone levels, which are regulated by the environment or the body, always change at the beginning of plant senescence. For instance, if the hormone auxin is artificially kept from having an effect on the plant, the plant lives longer than usual and experiences an unusually extended pattern of senescent transformation.

The study of the aging processes of insects displaying two different types of adaptive coloration yields useful conclusions: the aposematic, in which the bright markings act as a warning that the insect is poisonous or has a bad taste, and the procryptic, in which the patterns and colors allow the insect to conceal itself in its natural habitat. The two adaptation patterns have different optimal strategies for species survival:

the aposematics have longer post-reproductive survival, increasing their opportunity to condition predators, while the procryptics die out as soon as possible after completing reproduction, reducing the opportunity for predators to learn how to detect them. The saturniid moth family is home to both adaptations. Research has revealed that an enzyme system that regulates the amount of time spent in flight determines how long a species will survive after reproduction: aposematics fly less, save energy, and live longer, while procryptics fly more, exhaust themselves, and die sooner.

These examples show that senescence has an onset that is closely associated with the completion of the reproductive process and is governed by relatively simple enzymatic mechanisms that can be modified by natural selection in semelparous forms, in which full vigor and function are required until virtually the end of life. These kinds of targeted, genetically regulated senescence processes are examples of predetermined death.

The majority of vertebrates, most longer-lived insects,

crabs, spiders, cephalopod and gastropod mollusks, and perennial plants are classified as iteroparous forms. Iteroparous organisms, unlike semelparous forms, do not have to survive to the end of their reproductive phase in order to reproduce successfully. The average fraction of the reproductive span survived varies greatly between groups; for example, small rodents and birds in the wild typically only survive 10–20 percent of their potential lifetimes; large mammals such as whales, elephants, apes, and other mammals live 50–100 percent of their reproductive spans in the wild; and a small percentage even survive beyond reproductive age. Senescence in iteroparous forms develops gradually, and there is no indication of a particular systemic or environmental beginning mechanism. Senescence initially appears as a reduction in reproductive capacity. Reproductive capacity declines fairly early in species that reach a fixed body size, and it quickens with age. The number of eggs laid annually rises with age and body size in giant egg-laying reptiles, which reach sexual maturity at a relatively small size and continue to expand over a long reproductive career, but eventually level off and fall. In certain situations, the reproductive life span is less than the life span.

These parallels highlight the impact that population dynamics considerations have on the development of both reproductive and somatic senescence. It is evident that when the number of an individual's living progeny increases, their relative contribution to the rate of increase of the iteroparous population decreases. Additionally, as a person ages, their ability to procreate decreases. These data suggest that a maximum number of litters in a lifetime exists. The question of whether population dynamics influences result in the evolution of adaptive senescence patterns has been discussed by gerontologists for a while, but it hasn't been thoroughly studied yet.

There are certain indications that calorie restriction postpones reproductive senescence. This phenomenon can be accounted for, at least in part, by the advantageous impacts on the hypothalamus and pituitary gland that augment luteinizing hormone secretion, thereby regulating the activity of the gonads, or sex glands.

Variations in longevity and aging between species.

Some animal species have significantly different life spans. Among animals, the taxonomic stratification of longevity is evident. Although some little prosimians and New World monkeys have relatively limited life spans, primates are generally the group with the longest lifespans. The sciurid (squirrel-like) rodents can live up to three times longer than the murids, which are rodents that resemble mice.

Brain weight, body weight, and resting metabolic rate are the three characteristics that have independent relationships with life span. An equation representing the relationship between life span and these characteristics is $L = 5.5E\ 0.54S\ -0.34M\ -0.42$. Mammalian life span (L) is a function of metabolic rate (M) in calories per gram per hour, body weight (S), and brain weight (E) in grams. Regardless of body size or metabolic rate, the positive exponent for E (0.54) shows that there is a substantial positive correlation between mammal longevity and brain size.

If body weight and brain weight remain constant, the negative coefficient for metabolic rate suggests that life expectancy falls as the rate of living rises. The negative partial coefficient for body weight suggests that the high positive correlation between body weight and brain weight and its negative association with metabolic rate, rather than body size, is the cause of large animals' propensity to live longer lives. For birds, the same kind of relation of L to E, S, and M applies; however, despite their greater body temperatures and metabolic rates, birds tend to live longer than mammals of similar brain and body sizes. Compared to mammals of similar size, larger reptiles have longer lifespans, but because of their roughly ten-fold lower metabolic rates, they use less energy overall over their lifetimes. Greater lifetime energy outputs are found in more highly cephalized species, particularly primates, who have larger brain weights. For humans and domestic animals like cats and dogs, the total lifetime energy output per gram of tissue is approximately 1,200,000 and 400,000 calories, respectively.

For homeothermic mammals, or those with almost consistent body temperatures, the aforementioned relationships are valid. Because they can go into seasonal hibernation or daily torpor, heterothermic mammals can lower their metabolic rates by more than ten times. The most striking example are the insectivorous bats found in temperate climates; while they can live longer than 20 years, about 80 percent of that time is spent in deep torpor, meaning that their lifetime energy expenditures are no higher than those of other small mammals.

Arthropod species can live anywhere from a few days to several decades. The longer-living spiders and crustaceans are iteroparous, with yearly reproductive cycles, in contrast to the incredibly short-lived insects, which have a brief single reproductive phase.

The longevity gene inheritance

A comparison of the life tables of multiple inbred populations and some of their hybrids is used to evaluate the inheritance of longevity in animal populations, such as fruit flies and mice. Over forty inbred strains of mice have had sample populations' lifespans measured.

According to two investigations, roughly 20 percent of the variation in male mice's longevity is heritable, whereas about 30 percent of the variation in female mice's longevity is governed by genetics. The heritabilities of some physiological performances of domestic animals, including lifetime egg or milk production, are equivalent to these values. The rate of actuarial aging is indicated by the slope of the Gompertz function line. Variations in the rate of aging account for the majority of the differences in longevity between species, and these variations are reflected in variations in the Gompertz function's slope.

A comparison of life tables among strains of mice within the same species reveals that variations in age-independent hardiness parameters account for the majority of the strain variances. The parallel Gompertz functions demonstrate that if strains differ in hardiness, the less hardy have greater mortality rates by a constant multiple at all ages. First-generation (F1) hybrids of two inbred strains often have longer life spans than either parent.

Although the rates of the biochemical aging processes in hybrid and inbred mice have not been directly compared, life table comparisons suggest that hybrid vigor (heterosis) is a gain in age-independent vigor rather than a decrease in the pace of aging.

A significant portion of the variance in survival duration amongst mouse strains can be attributed to variations in genetic susceptibility to particular illnesses. Deciding how much of these genetic influences there are on aging is a key challenge in the field of gerontology.

It is more challenging to study how people inherit their longer lifespans since socioeconomic status and other environmental factors can create erroneous associations between closely related individuals. Many studies have been published, the majority of which indicate that there is some heredity in terms of lifespan or vulnerability to serious illnesses like cancer and heart disease. The degree to which human longevity is heritable is a topic of debate, but there is substantial evidence that genetics plays a role in the development of coronary heart disease and related disorders, as well as the tendency for monozygotic (genetically identical) twins to live longer than like-sex dizygotic (genetically different, fraternal) twins.

Senescence in Mammals

alterations in exercise, metabolism, and body composition

After reaching physical maturity, the lean body mass—which is made up of the skeletal muscles and all other cellular tissues—decreases gradually until it reaches severe old age, at which point it may be as low as two-thirds of its youthful value. However, as people age, their body weight often rises because they lose less lean body mass and more stored fat and water in their bodies. The proportion of extracellular fluid steadily decreases during fetal and postnatal development before increasing with age in adulthood. Therefore, aging causes all tissues—including the skin—to become increasingly water-laden, despite appearances to the contrary. Adults' voluntary (striated) muscular tissue mass gradually decreases over time, depending in part on their physical exercise habits.

Research suggests that atrophy and lack of usage, rather than the loss of muscle fibers, account for a significant portion of the age-related loss of muscle mass.

The level of total metabolic activity decreases in tandem with the loss of lean body mass. The highest level of basal metabolism occurs during the fastest possible bulk increase. After that, it declines more slowly until physical maturity is reached. Over a three-year period, the sluggish phase of reduction in rats amounts to approximately 20 percent. Even though less heat is produced, the body's internal temperature is preserved because there is less blood flow through the skin, which reduces heat loss. Therefore, the "cooling of the blood" that comes with aging does not happen to the extent that one may assume based on a drop in skin temperature. Though it varies greatly across different animals, the amount of voluntary physical activity, like jogging on an exercise wheel, usually declines with age.

Humans are more susceptible to developing metabolic diseases such as type II diabetes mellitus, hyperlipidemia (high blood levels of lipids), arteriosclerosis (hardening of the arteries), and hypertension (high blood pressure) as a result of general aging-related changes in metabolism that cause increased fat deposition and decreased muscle mass. In certain individuals, these diseases may manifest together, leading to the development of a disorder referred to as metabolic syndrome.

Age also causes a decrease in ghrelin, a hormone that increases food intake and is mostly produced and secreted by the gastrointestinal mucosa in humans. Because the gastric mucosa is less functional as we age, there is a decrease in circulating ghrelin levels. This decrease is believed to be connected to the anorexia and appetite loss that are frequently seen in elderly adults.

Modifications to the structural tissues

Collagen and elastin are two types of fibrous protein molecules that are essential to the structural integrity of vertebrates. Collagen is a protein present in tendons, skin, and bones that makes up about one-third of all body proteins.

Upon initial synthesis by fibroblast cells, collagen exists in a soluble and delicate form known as tropocollagen. This soluble collagen eventually transforms into an insoluble, more stable version that can stay in the tissues of an animal for the majority of its life. The ratio of insoluble to soluble collagen rises with age because the rate of synthesis of collagen is high in youth and decreases throughout adulthood. Then, as we age, insoluble collagen accumulates because its synthesis outpaces its clearance, a process similar to that of the crystalline lens in our eyes, another fibrous tissue. The quantity of cross-links inside and between collagen molecules rises with age, resulting in crystallinity and rigidity, which are mirrored in the overall stiffness of the body. Additionally, there is a reduction in the relative quantity of a mucopolysaccharide, or the mixture of a protein and a carbohydrate, in ground material; the hexosamine-collagen ratio, a measure of this, has been studied as a potential indicator of individual variations in the pace of aging.

Reduced tissue permeability to dissolved nutrients, hormones, and antibody molecules is a significant effect of these alterations.

Collagen ages more quickly in animals with higher metabolic activity than in rats fed a complete meal; rats kept on low-calorie diets had younger-looking collagen than rats of the same age fed a full diet.

The chemical that gives blood vessel walls their suppleness is called elastin. Vascular elasticity gradually declines with age, most likely as a result of elastin molecule breakage.

Collagen cross-links are chemically similar to cross-links seen in skins that have been tanned to leather. Due to these similarities, theories have been raised suggesting that substances that prevent tanning's cross-linking will slow down aging.

Loss and replacement of tissue cells

Whether or not tissue cell renewal occurs continuously divides the body's tissues into two categories. Nonrenewal tissues, like voluntary muscles and nerves, are at one extreme of the spectrum.

After a particular growth stage, very few new cells can be formed in these tissues, at least not in mammals. On the other hand, some cell types in renewal tissues, like the blood and intestinal epithelium, only survive a few days or a week and need to be replaced hundreds of times over the life of even a short-lived animal, like the rat. Many organs, including the skin, liver, and endocrine system, fall between these ranges since their cell replacement cycles in humans can last anywhere from a few weeks to many years.

Since it is possible to count all of the fibers in the nerve trunk, studying a peripheral nerve is convenient. Rats, cats, and people have all had their cervical and thoracic spinal nerve roots treated in this way. Between the ages of 30 and 90, there is a roughly 20% reduction in the number of nerve fibers in the human ventral and dorsal spinal roots. However, the findings do not consistently show that the number of spinal root fibers decreases with age in the cat, rat, or mouse.

In humans, the number of optic nerve fibers, which support vision, declines at a pace almost equal to that of olfactory nerve fibers, which support smell, by the age of 90, to around 25% of the total number present at birth.

Human age causes a notable reduction in the number of live cells in the cerebral cortex of the brain. Rat and human cerebellar cortex degradation with age is similar to that of the cerebral cortex. Aging leaves less of an evident impression on other areas of the brain.

In summary, there is a tendency for the upper and more recently formed nervous system levels to lose their youthfulness more severely than other regions, like the spinal cord and brainstem. It is currently unknown how much of the death of brain cells is caused by internal brain disorders and how much is due to external factors like deteriorating blood circulation. Neuroglia, the tiny cells that surround neurons, are crucial for the nourishment and upkeep of nerve cells, or neurons, in the central nervous system.

Although it appears that the total number of these cells does not diminish with age, some of the microscopic alterations observed in elderly people's neurons are comparable to those brought on by physical or dietary exhaustion.

It has been demonstrated that following a measles episode, the virus stays in the host's body for the duration of their life and sporadically causes a rapidly worsening cerebral cortex degeneration. Individual variations in the onset of senility in humans may also be caused by this virus or other inapparent viruses.

A population of proliferative cells, which are still able to divide, and a population of mature cells, which are produced by the proliferative cells and have a shorter lifespan, usually make up the renewal tissues. Each regeneration tissue contains one or more channels of feedback control to adapt production to demand. This is because the creation of cells needs to balance the continuous loss and also swiftly compensate for unexpected losses brought on by damage or disease.

Rejuvenation tissues age in a variety of ways, including as a reduction in the quantity of proliferative cells, a slowing down of cell division, and a diminished receptiveness to feedback signals. Though these factors do not appreciably alter the blood-forming tissues of mice, aging does cause a deficit in these tissues because older mice have a markedly diminished capacity to respond to repeated or harsh demands.

In reaction to injury, the intact skin, like all regeneration tissues, can temporarily increase its rate of cell creation by a significant amount. However, the skin's cell turnover time is several weeks. As one ages, the rate of wound healing slows down; initially, it happens quickly.

The loss of focus on both near and far objects is one of the most common and noticeable effects of aging. A reduction in the flexibility of the lens and a weakening of the ciliary muscle of the eye are contributing factors to this loss of visual accommodation. But the lens grows throughout life at a pace that decreases with age, which is another contributing factor.

This expansion is the outcome of epithelial cells continuously dividing close to the lens's hypothetical midline, producing new cells that develop into the precisely aligned lens fibers. The fibers are fixed in place once they are created.

The stem cell is a key component of the renewal mechanism. Under circumstances of heightened demand, these cells—which may typically divide slowly throughout their lives—enter a compensatory proliferative phase in which they divide quickly. In young people, the stem cell population in blood-forming tissue is highly responsive to injury, but as one ages, this capacity decreases. The loss of blood-forming stem cells has been linked to an increased risk of anemia with aging and a decreased ability to react to blood loss. There is uncertainty regarding the identities of stem cell groups in different proliferative tissues. Particularly in the intestinal mucosa, there is a high rate of cell division without any discernible reserve population of stem cells.

Neurological and endocrine system aging

The brain experiences both adaptability and degeneration as it ages. The brain receives less blood as neurons shrink and die. Reduced oxygen delivery to tissues, such as the brain and eyes, may arise from the latter. As we age, our eyes' capacity to dark-adapt—that is, to become more sensitive in low light—decreases; nevertheless, breathing pure oxygen can somewhat compensate for this loss. In older adults, breathing oxygen has also been demonstrated to aid a variety of brain processes. Protein synthesis is a step in the formation of a memory trace, which is a set of connections in the brain linked to memory. Age-related decreased stimulation of protein synthesis, such as from reduced oxygen intake, may contribute to memory and learning deficiencies in the elderly. However, the aging brain also creates new synapses, or connections between neurons, which helps to make up for the loss of neurons at the same time that they are degenerating.

The endocrine system ages generally in such a way that the cells that were formerly highly responsive to hormones become less so.

Cyclic adenosine monophosphate (AMP), a typical cell component, is believed to be a messenger of hormonal information across cell membranes. It could be able to pinpoint the precise locations in the membrane or inside the cell where communication breaks down.

The pituitary gland influences both the neurological and endocrine systems due to its connection to both systems. Aging reduces the pituitary gland's sensitivity to growth hormone-releasing hormone. Growth hormone release is subsequently inhibited as a result, which has an impact on the general rate and effectiveness of metabolic processes.

Aging's internal and external causes

agents in the external environment

radiation that ionizes

It has been established that ionizing radiation, such as X-rays, shortens the life span of numerous animals, including dogs, rats, mice, hamsters, and guinea pigs. Certain diseases, including leukemia, may become more common disproportionately following radiation, with age and gender influencing how much more common they become.

The comparison of the life spans of the exposed and control groups demonstrates the irreversible nature of radiation damage. Similar to a historically older, unirradiated population, an irradiated population eventually dies. Individuals in a population who receive a single dose of gamma or X-rays in their early adult years pass away from the same illnesses that affect the unirradiated control group, but they do so months or even years sooner.

The process of mortality is accelerated by low-dose continuous radiation exposure throughout life, with daily doses ranging from a thousandth to a tenth of the dosage that would cause immediate death. Extensive research on animals and cultured cells indicates that high radiation dosages cause lethal chromosomal rearrangements in the proliferating cell population. Although these aberrations also get worse with age, they don't seem to have as much of an impact on aging naturally. Chromosome aberrations become comparatively less significant than other consequences at low radiation doses, and the primary radiation damage in these settings may be more closely associated with the aging lesion.

Even in the long-lived human species, background radiation from cosmic rays and natural radioactivity in the body, which largely comes from radioactive potassium and radium, do not significantly contribute to aging. However, their contribution to the incidence of cancer is negligible. Nuclear weapon test fallout radiation is less than 1% of background radiation, while medical radiation doses to the body are only a small portion of background levels. Both sources contribute proportionately to the development of cancer.

The temperature

Fish, flour beetles, fruit flies, and other species that are temperature-variable—or poikilothermic—live longer in lower environmental temperature ranges. The rate-of-living hypothesis, which, to put it simply, maintains that an organism's life span is based on some key ingredient that gets depleted more quickly at higher temperatures, was born out of these facts. Nevertheless, a thorough examination of the temperature-longevity relationship data reveals that the rate-of-living hypothesis is insufficient in its original form.

Experiments where fruit flies were housed at one temperature for a portion of their lives and at a different temperature for the rest provide the most compelling data. Although the rate-of-living hypothesis cannot explain the data, a plausible theory has not yet emerged to replace it. An essential component that has not yet received enough consideration is the relationship between temperature and metabolic efficiency. It has been found that the energy cost of the biosynthetic processes under study increases at higher or lower temperatures and is negligible at an intermediate temperature within the range to which the species is adapted. A similar phenomenon pertains to longevity: fruit flies experience the least amount of aging per calorie at an intermediate temperature because their lifelong energy expenditure is highest there.

The extent to which heat degradation (thermal denaturation) of proteins causes aging is a matter of debate. The primary cause of thermal denaturation is primarily the disruption of molecular folding, which necessitates the breaking of several low-energy bonds.

It doesn't appear to be a major cause of aging. It's still possible that uncommon occurrences like mutations could result from thermal denaturation to a considerable extent. Since there is a correlation between short life spans in shorter-lived species and high metabolisms, which raise core temperatures, research has shown that humans might live longer if their body temperatures were lower. An approximate 20 percent increase in life span was linked to a drop in body temperature of 0.5 °C (0.9 °F) in a study of mice that were genetically modified to have a lower-than-normal core body temperature.

Indications of Early Aging

Everybody ages, but premature aging occurs when aging occurs more quickly than it ought to. Usually, lifestyle and environmental variables are the root causes. The most prevalent indications of early aging are wrinkles, age spots, dryness, and a loss of skin tone. Adopting a healthy lifestyle can help halt and avoid additional premature aging.

Section Four

Potential Reasons

Why do people age too soon?

Premature aging is typically caused by preventable and controllable conditions. We refer to this as extrinsic aging.

Your skin is where the majority of early-aging symptoms appear. As we age, our skin changes. When they first manifest earlier in life, environmental or lifestyle factors are typically to blame.

Premature aging is primarily caused by exposure to light. Numerous skin issues are caused by sun exposure. Your skin ages faster from UV light and sunshine exposure than it would from natural aging. Ninety percent of the noticeable alterations to your skin are caused by this outcome, which is known as photoaging. UV rays harm skin cells, which causes early alterations like age spots.

The danger of skin cancer is also raised by this sun exposure.

The remaining 10% of skin alterations are caused by high-energy visual (HEV) and infrared light. Blue light, or HEV light, is emitted by electronic gadgets such as cellphones and the sun. Despite being invisible, infrared light is frequently perceived as heat. These types of light have an impact on skin elasticity and collagen but do not raise the risk of skin cancer.

Other elements of the environment or way of life that contribute to early aging include:

Smoking: The toxins in nicotine change your body's cells when you smoke. Your skin's collagen and elastic fibers are broken down by these toxins, which causes sagging, wrinkles, and a hollow, gaunt face.

Unhealthy diet: A few studies suggest that diets heavy in refined carbs or sugar can hasten the aging process. Conversely, diets rich in fruits and vegetables can help avert premature aging of the skin.

Alcohol: Excessive alcohol consumption can cause skin damage and dehydration, which can result in early indications of aging.

Insufficient or poor sleep: Research indicates that sleep deprivation accelerates the aging process of cells.

Stress: The stress hormone cortisol is released by the brain in response to stress. Hyaluronan synthase and collagen are two components that keep your skin looking youthful and plump, and cortisol inhibits both of them.

Rarely, some illnesses can result in early aging symptoms.

Bloom's syndrome.

Type III or type I Cockayne syndrome.

Hutchinson-Gilford syndrome of progeria.

Mandibuloacral dysplasia with type A lipodystrophy.

Rothmund-Thomson syndrome.

Seip syndrome.

Werner syndrome.

Care and treatment

What steps can I take to avoid or halt aging too soon?

As lifestyle and environmental factors frequently contribute to early aging, adopting healthy daily practices can help prevent it. Here's how to stop premature aging if you currently exhibit symptoms and keep them from growing worse:

Steer clear of the sun. Take precautions against sun damage. Throughout the year, even if you intend to be in the shade, wear sunscreen. Choose UV protection with at least SPF 30 or above at all times. Put on protection gear, such as sunglasses and a hat. Use self-tanning products instead of tanning booths.

Give up smoking. If you smoke, give it up as soon as you can. If you need assistance stopping, speak with your healthcare professional.

Consume more fruits and vegetables because a balanced diet can prevent aging prematurely. Refined carbs and sugar should be consumed in moderation.

Reducing your alcohol intake can help avoid further harm to your skin, as alcohol accelerates the aging process of your skin.

Exercise: Engaging in regular physical activity strengthens your immune system and circulatory system, all of which support good aging.

Take good care of your skin by cleansing it once a day to get rid of debris, makeup, perspiration, and other irritating elements. Avoid using harsh skin care products with strong perfumes or high pH levels. To avoid dryness and itching, moisturize your skin every day.

Reduce your stress levels. Make an effort to live a life free of as much stress as you can. For the stressors you are unable to avoid, discover constructive coping mechanisms (such as exercise or meditation).

Boost the quantity and quality of your sleep. Your body's cells will age more quickly if you get less than seven hours of sleep.

How can I stop myself from aging too soon?

Healthy living is the key to prevention in order to avoid premature aging. However, these therapies can help reverse signs of premature aging if they are bothering you:

Fillers for the skin.

Facelift.

Regeneration and resurfacing of the face.

Skin resurfacing with lasers.

Be aware that while these treatments might improve the appearance of premature aging, they won't address the underlying cause of the condition.

When to Make a Doctor's Appointment

When should I visit my doctor if I notice any early-aging symptoms?

If symptoms of early aging increase quickly, are painful or uncomfortable, or appear suddenly, speak with your healthcare professional.

A message from the Cleveland Clinic

Any stage of adulthood might experience signs of premature aging, which are typically brought on by lifestyle or environmental factors. Rare syndromes can sometimes lead to early aging. Premature aging can be prevented or reversed by exercising, quitting smoking, eating a well-balanced diet, and protecting your skin from the sun. See your doctor about possible therapies if premature aging continues or starts to affect you.

Section Five

The younger for life initiative

A Handbook for Youth: How to Live Your Life

As a high school student, I'm reminded all the time to consider my options for a profession and other aspects of my life. I absolutely get extreme pressure from my parents and professors to solve problems right away. I don't want to make a mistake now since I'm young and spoil my future. I am aware of my preferences and hobbies, but for some reason, every time I read about a profession that relates to those things, I get the feeling that I wouldn't enjoy it.

What to do with your future is a really difficult decision to make! Now that I'm older and still working things out, I can't really advise this young woman what to do because her parents might not appreciate that very much.

But I can share with her what I've learned from looking back on my life and what I would tell my own children (I have a 14-year-old girl and a 21-year-old son who are both my kids).

That's what I would say.

It is impossible to predict the future. Even young individuals who aspire to be doctors, lawyers, research scientists, singers, or other professions are unsure about what the future holds. They seem a little misguided, if they are certain at all. While some people may accomplish everything they set out to do, you never know if you're one of those people. Life rarely goes as planned. Things happen that have the power to alter you, your prospects, and the course of history. For example, there was no such thing as a Twitter account, Google account, or Amazon account when I was a teenager. Neither did the blogger for Zen Habits.

What do you do if you are unable to predict the future? Keep your eyes off the future.

Pay attention to what you can accomplish today that will benefit you in the future, regardless of what it holds. Produce things. Construct things. Acquire abilities. Take on adventures. Make friends. These items will be beneficial in the future.

Become adept at handling discomfort. Developing the ability to tolerate some discomfort is one of the most crucial abilities you can acquire. The greatest things in life are frequently challenging, and you will miss out if you avoid hardship and discomfort. You'll lead a secure existence.

Acquiring knowledge is challenging. It takes work to build anything truly amazing. Book writing is difficult. Marriage is challenging. It's difficult to run an ultramarathon. They're all quite wonderful.

You can accomplish anything if you get skilled at this. Since launching a business is difficult and uncomfortable, you can do it, whereas you couldn't if you're terrified of discomfort.

How can you improve at this? Now, intentionally do activities that are difficult and uncomfortable.

But begin with modest dosages. Even if it's difficult, try doing some light exercise for a few minutes at a time, increasing by one minute about every few days. Attempt blogging or daily meditation. Push yourself a little bit harder when you find yourself avoiding discomfort (within reasonable and acceptable bounds, of course).

Develop your ability to handle ambiguity. Living well in the unknown is a similar ability. For instance, launching a business is an incredible endeavor, but if you're scared of the unknown, you won't undertake it. You can't predict the future, so if you try to predict it, you'll miss out on amazing chances, businesses, and projects.

You'll be open to a lot more options, though, if you can accept not knowing. Study up on uncertainty.

If you thrive in discomfort and uncertainty, you could write a book, launch a business, teach English abroad, travel the world and live cheaply while blogging about it, learn to program and make your own software, work for a startup, launch an online magazine with other talented young writers, and much more.

While all of these things seem fantastic, you have to be able to tolerate discomfort and uncertainty.

If you've honed these abilities, you'll be prepared for any such opportunities.

Get rid of distractions and put off tasks. If you can't get over the common issues of procrastination and distraction, none of this will matter. Because you're adept at handling uncertainty and pain, you might grab a chance, but you might miss it because you're too preoccupied with social media and TV.

As procrastination and distraction are really just strategies for avoiding discomfort, you'll be far ahead of most people if you can master them. However, there are certain exercises you can do; find out more here.

Discover more about your mental state. Most individuals are unaware of how much fear governs them. When they divert themselves or justify doing things they promised themselves they wouldn't do, they are unaware of it. Changing mental habits is difficult because you are not always aware of what is happening inside your head.

Gain knowledge about the functioning of your mind, and you'll excel in all of these areas. Blogging and meditation are the finest methods. When you meditate (see how to do it), you can observe how your mind wanders, tries to comfort itself, and rationalizes itself. Blogging forces you to take stock of your life experiences and the lessons you've learned. I suggest it to all young people as an excellent instrument for personal development.

Earn a little cash. Although I don't think money is all that significant, it is not easy to make money. To be hired or have someone purchase your goods or services, you must convince them of your worth. This requires you to come up with a compelling case for your credibility. You must earn the right to be worthy. To get people to want to buy from or hire you, you also need to learn how to express that to them. This applies to selling cookies door-to-door, apps in the Apple Store, and applying for jobs as cashiers. And practice makes perfect.

During my high school years, I held jobs as a bank clerk and a freelance sports writer, both of which were beneficial experiences for me.

A piece of advice is to save aside money for emergencies, then begin investing your earnings in index funds to see them rise over time.

Construct a little object. The majority of individuals waste their time on unimportant stuff like TV, video games, social networking, and news reading. A year of that, and you have nothing to show for it. However, if you draw something every day, begin coding a web application, start a regularly updated blog or video channel, or begin developing a cookie company, you'll have something amazing at the end of a year. also a few fresh abilities. Something that most people are not able to build, but you can point to and say, "I built that."

If at all feasible, start small and expand it each day. It appreciates in value over time, much like investing your money.

Develop credibility. The greatest concern for anyone hiring a young person is that they may not be reliable.

That they'll miss deadlines, arrive late, and fabricate an excuse. An individual with a well-established reputation over time may be far more reliable and have a higher chance of getting employed. Develop your reliability by being a kind person, being punctual, being honest, owning up to mistakes but correcting them, and doing your best to complete tasks on time.

Doing so will help you establish a reputation and gain referrals from others, which is the ideal approach to finding employment or attracting investors.

Prepare yourself for opportunities. If you do all of the above, or at least most of it, you'll be wonderful. You will be far, far ahead of the majority of others in your age group. If you keep your eyes open, possibilities will present themselves to you, such as the possibility to submit a new script, construct something with someone, learn something new and turn it into a business, or get a job.

You need to be prepared to take advantage of these possibilities when they present themselves. One benefit of being young is that you can afford to take chances. And make your own if none are available.

Ultimately, the underlying concept behind all of this is that you can never know what you will do with your life at this point because you never know who you will become, what you will be capable of, what you will be passionate about, who you will meet, what chances you will have, or the state of the world. You are aware, nevertheless, that you are capable of everything you set your mind to.

Get ready by mastering discomfort and uncertainty, constructing things, learning about your thinking, developing trust, and beating procrastination.

You can ignore all of this and lead a boring, safe life. Alternatively, you may begin right now and experience what life has to offer.

Finally, how do you respond to pressure from parents and teachers to solve problems on your own? Inform them that you intend to become an entrepreneur, launch your own company, and conquer the globe. You'll be ready for any career if you prepare for it.

Being young is synonymous with the future, change, and advancement. In the end, being youthful means overcoming obstacles and reclaiming or creating a space for complete development in the future.

It entails being the engine of society and transforming obstacles into chances and answers.

We commemorate "Youth Engagement for Global Action," a slogan that aims to emphasize the ways in which young people interact at the local, national, and international levels, today on International Youth Day 2020. We also honor their visions and choices.

Both local problems and global ones, such as the coronavirus epidemic and climate change, will have an impact on the future. It's time to find out how much this impacts the younger generation and to propose remedies. The largest generation in history is comprised of those between the ages of 14 and 29.

We spoke with a number of young Cubans to learn about their aspirations and their places in society, both as members of the populace and as individuals. These young people observe society from their unique perspective and consider ways to imbue it with their own uniqueness. They were given two questions to answer and were asked to share their answers.

What do you believe modern youth should be doing? What actions are you taking in your role to support youth?

Magdany Acosta Gallardo, eighteen

Young people are not only our nation's future; we are also one of the primary forces driving social advancement and change. We also have a significant impact on economic growth. We form a lot of social connections and a distinct personality throughout this phase of our lives, which sets us apart as a new generation. How we think and behave now will determine what we do as adults.

The age of Yaicelín Palma Tejas is 27.

Teenagers have only one role in life, and it is the same role they have always played. It stays the same since their job is to make everything better than it was and to bring happiness and vitality to everything.

As a journalist, I believe that one way I can support young people is by emphasizing our ability to effect change. I support all calls for liberation and autonomy as a young citizen because these are issues that affect people everywhere.

22-year-old Carlos Alejandro Sánchez

I believe that regardless of the society they live in, youth today are extremely important. Whether we realize it or not, we are the ones changing our reality—whether it is at work, at school, or in other settings—by bringing fresh perspectives to routine tasks. It is our duty to push for social change and to effectively voice our opinions in society.

Undoubtedly, having the chance to appear on radio or television every day, along with my widespread presence on social media, has made it easier for me to share my ideas and thoughts with a far larger audience than I would have otherwise been able to. I'm really glad that I can use my words and deeds to positively impact my generation and others. I've been able to demonstrate that no matter how young you are, if you want something and are prepared to fight for it, you can achieve it since everything in life is about perseverance and attitude. For instance, anchoring a news program or a show focused on a young audience is a great responsibility.

25-year-old Roxana Broche

The youth are the backbone of the community and a symbol of intergenerational transition. Although it has been said a lot, young people are actually the ones who are responsible for leaving a legacy.

I believe that, as an actress, I can use my personal and professional experiences to uplift and support young people without overdoing the message. The more life experiences one shares, the more knowledge they may impart, and sharing knowledge for the benefit of others is, in my opinion, a crucial component.

Anthony Bravo, a 20-year-old

As a young singer, I am fortunate to have a voice, but with that comes great responsibility. For this reason, my current work focuses on spreading positive messages and attempting to model behaviors that foster personal development. These efforts ultimately propel a collective creation grounded in values that prioritize the well-being of society over the well-being of individuals. Ensuring our personal well-being is the finest approach to making a constructive contribution to the community; after all, humanism begins at home.

I've made it my mission to represent concepts that I believe are beneficial through my music and lyrics, as well as through my work as a design student and an active member of our nation. My time and ideas have been dedicated to serving my generation.

Luis Daniel Carralero del Riego. 16 years old

Our age-appropriate duty in the world is to perform some crucial tasks for our society before developing into responsible, time-bound adults. For instance, in the protracted battle against some people's inaction to stop global warming, young people are taking the lead and immobilizing the entire world. We have demonstrated our ability to provide a brighter future and our willingness to overcome all obstacles in order to do so.

27-year-old Leslie Alonso Figueroa

It is the challenge of the youth to strive for a just world without forgetting the past. Among the obstacles to be overcome are racism, chauvinism by men, gender violence, and phobias and discrimination.

Young people from all walks of life—whether they be from the job, school, or community—must unite in the ultimate goal of establishing societies of rights, with everyone's support and benefit.

The issues facing children around the world are issues that affect us as well, which makes my work as a professor and communicator very challenging. We all live and dwell in the same environment, where factors like the new coronavirus and climate change drive us to reconsider our approaches and roles in order to create the future we require.

Harold Naranjo, Twenty-One

In my view, today's youth have an extremely important role to play. While some may not have a clear purpose in life, I'm sure that many are able to realize their ambitions through acting, dancing, singing, and other artistic endeavors. That's all I see in a program like Center A+ Espacios Adolescentes, which I consider fortunate to be a part of and which offers the chance to explore creative capacities!

In my situation, I was able to address the various concerns of boys and girls who could relate to the content by hosting radio shows because we cover relevant subjects and teach useful skills that help teens, young adults, and families in general create the society we want.

Linda Milian Betancourt. 16 years old

The youth demographic is a valuable asset to society, as they are catalysts for social transformation, economic advancement, and development.

Section Six

How to take care of your age

You may age gracefully from the inside out by using these strategies.

Treat your skin with kindness. The largest organ in your body is your skin.

Work out. ...

Take care of your diet.

Mental well-being is important.

Continue your physical activity.

Reduce your tension.

Give up drinking alcohol and stop smoking.

Make time to go to sleep.

How to Enjoy Your Older Years to the Fullest

What does gentle aging entail?

There are always at least a few magazine articles about how to look younger when you are in the checkout line. There's so much more to aging healthily, even though some wrinkles and sagging are what most people fear.

Living your best life and being in good enough physical and mental health to appreciate it are the keys to aging gracefully, not attempting to look like a twentysomething. Like a bottle of wine, you can get better with age with the appropriate care.

Continue reading to learn what to do and what not to do in your endeavor to age gracefully.

Advice on how to age gracefully

You may age gracefully from the inside out by using these strategies.

1. **Treat your skin with kindness**.

The largest organ in your body is your skin. It may better shield your body from the weather, control body temperature, and provide feeling if you take good care of it.

To keep it looking and working at its best:

When you're outside, put on protective clothes and sunscreen.

Get screened for skin cancer every year.

When it comes to your anti-aging skin care regimen, stick to moderate products.

Remain hydrated.

2. Work out

Frequent exercise helps you maintain your mobility for a longer period of time and dramatically reduces your risk of diseases like cancer and heart disease. In addition, exercise enhances mood, skin and bone health, sleep quality, and stress reduction.

Adults are advised to undertake the following by the Department of Health and Human Services (trusted source):

1.25 to 2.5 hours of vigorous-intensity aerobic exercise per week, 2.5 to 5 hours of moderate-intensity exercise per week, or a mix of the two.

Two or more days a week, engaging in moderately intense muscle-strengthening exercises that target all main muscle groups.

Here are a few instances of aerobic exercise:

Strolling

Swimming

Dancing

Riding

Resistance bands, or weights, can be used for activities that strengthen bones and muscles.

In addition to cardiovascular and muscle-strengthening workouts, older people should prioritize balance-training activities.

3. Be mindful of your diet.

Eating a healthy diet is the key to aging gracefully. According to the Dietary Guidelines for Americans (Trusted Source), you should eat:

fruits and vegetables in tinned, frozen, or fresh form

lean protein foods like beans and fish

a minimum of three ounces of whole-grain breads, rice, pasta, or cereal per day.

Three servings of dairy products that are low in fat or fat-free, including vitamin D-fortified milk, yogurt, or cheese.

Good fats

For cooking, utilize oils rather than solid fats. Avoid refined sweets, processed meals, and foods high in harmful fats.

Reduce your intake of salt as well if you want to lower your blood pressure.

4. It matters for mental health.

Living a joyful and stress-free life contributes significantly to aging well.

To maintain a positive attitude:

Spend time with your loved ones and friends. Strong social networks and meaningful interactions enhance longevity and promote both physical and mental health.

Remember your furry family members; studies have shown that owning a pet lowers blood pressure and stress levels, as well as reduces loneliness and improves mood.

Recognize your age. Research suggests that those with a positive outlook on aging have longer lifespans and may heal from disabilities more effectively.

Understanding that aging is inevitable can have a profound impact.

Engage in activities you find enjoyable. Spending time doing things you enjoy can only increase your level of happiness. Whatever makes you happy, do it: take up a new activity, volunteer, or spend time in nature.

5. Continue to be active.

A sedentary lifestyle is associated with a higher risk of chronic illness and premature death, according to numerous studies (trusted source).

Taking vacations, joining group exercise programs, and going on walks and treks are a few ways to keep active.

6. Reduce your anxiety.

Stress has a wide range of negative impacts on your body, from wrinkles and early aging to an increased chance of heart disease.

Many tried-and-true methods exist for reducing stress, such as:

Utilizing methods of relaxation, including yoga, breathing exercises, and meditation.

Working out

Obtaining enough rest

Conversing with a friend

7. **Give up smoking and cut back on drinking.**

It has been demonstrated that drinking alcohol and smoking both accelerate aging and raise the risk of disease.

Although giving up smoking is difficult, there are tools available to support you in your efforts. Consult a physician for advice on quitting.

To reduce your risk of illness, stick to the suggested source quantity when it comes to drinking. That equates to one drink for women and two for men each day.

8. **Make time to go to sleep**.

You need quality sleep for both your physical and emotional well-being. It affects the condition of your skin as well.

Your age determines the amount of sleep you require. Aim for seven to eight hours of sleep every night for those over the age of 18.

Sleeping sufficiently has been demonstrated to:

Reduce the chance of stroke and heart disease.

Lessen depression and stress.

Reduce the likelihood of obesity.

Lessen the inflammatory response.

Enhance concentration and focus.

9. Discover new interests.

Throughout your life, discovering new and fulfilling interests can help you stay engaged and have a sense of purpose.

Research from a reputable source indicates that people who participate in hobbies, leisure activities, and social gatherings live longer, are happier, and have less depression.

10.   Engage in mindfulness exercises.

Acceptance and present-focused living are key components of mindfulness. Being aware offers several scientifically supported health advantages that can improve your aging process, such as:

Enhanced concentration

Improved recall

Reduce tension

Enhanced emotional response

Contentment in relationships

Heightened immunity

Try these to cultivate mindfulness:

Meditation

Yoga

Tai Chi

Painting

## 11.	Sip a lot of water.

Getting adequate water enhances your energy and cognitive performance, as well as helping you stay regular. It's also been demonstrated by trusted sources to improve skin health and lessen aging symptoms.

Your recommended water intake is based on:

You're thirsty

Your degree of activity

the frequency of your bowel movements and urination

the amount of perspiration you produce.

What gender are you?

If you are unsure or worried about how much water you are consuming, consult a physician.

12.   Observe oral hygiene.

In addition to making your smile look older, not taking proper care of your teeth increases your risk of developing gum disease, which has been connected to bacterial pneumonia, heart attacks, and strokes.

Regular dental visits are essential in addition to good oral hygiene.

A dentist can identify symptoms of infections, cancer, malnutrition, and other disorders like diabetes, according to the American Dental Association. They advise using a mouth rinse, brushing twice a day, and flossing once a day.

13.   Visit a physician on a regular basis.

Regular medical checkups can assist the physician in identifying issues early on, or even before they arise. Your age, way of life, medical history, and current ailments all influence how frequently you visit the doctor.

As you get older, find out from your doctor how frequently you should get checkups and screenings. Additionally, consult a physician whenever you have unsettling symptoms.

Where to look for assistance

Even though growing older is a natural part of life, some people find it challenging to adapt to these changes.

It's critical to get help if you're experiencing health concerns, finding it difficult to embrace aging, or fearing that you're not aging gracefully.

Speak with a trusted person, like a member of your family or a close friend. You can also get professional assistance from a physician or counselor.

Being happy and healthy is more important for graceful aging than avoiding wrinkles.

Keep up a healthy lifestyle, spend time with the people you care about, and engage in activities that make you happy.

It's normal to be concerned about the difficulties that aging may present, so don't be afraid to voice your worries to someone.

Eight Superfoods to Help You Look Younger

The organ's unsung hero is the skin. The first organ in your body to reveal interior issues is your skin. Your body's greatest organ, your skin, will express gratitude if you have given it a balanced diet rich in antioxidants, good fats, water, vitamins, and other micronutrients.

Since internal factors contribute to skin aging, starting with your food is important. Naturally, eating a healthy diet is the most important way to prevent skin aging, but you should also take other lifestyle variables like sunscreen protection and skin care routines into account. Consuming foods high in vitamins and minerals is crucial for reversing the effects of aging.

The key ingredients of anti-aging meals are natural collagen boosters, ellagic acid, and a variety of vitamins. The middle layer of your skin contains collagen, which gives your skin a plump and full appearance. Collagen levels decrease with age, yet consuming a healthy diet naturally makes your skin seem more radiant. Vitamin C-rich foods can help lessen the appearance of aging skin. These are the top foods that prevent wrinkles and promote collagen and moisture for skin that looks younger and healthier.

1. Avocados

The most delicious and nutrient-dense fruit we have is the avocado. Monounsaturated and polyunsaturated fats found in avocados can nourish your skin and keep it from becoming dry. In order to maintain the health of your immune system, it also has anti-inflammatory properties. According to studies, the fruit's lutein and zeaxanthin may help shield your skin from UV-ray damage. Additionally, it is a great source of vitamins A, B, C, E, and K, which make your skin seem beautiful and glow.

Avocados can be used to make nutritious pudding or added to salads.

2. Broccoli

Broccoli has a ton of anti-aging and anti-inflammatory qualities! It has high levels of vitamin K and C, which are the finest antioxidants for preventing wrinkles. Your skin's support structure, collagen, is synthesized by your body using vitamin C. For the best benefits, try eating broccoli, either raw or steamed. It can be included in soups or salads. It also contains a lot of calcium and fiber.

3. Nuts

Nuts are a rich source of minerals, vitamins E, proteins, vital oils, and antioxidants. Walnuts and almonds are excellent sources of vitamin E, which helps shield your skin from the sun's UV rays. Additionally, vitamin E strengthens and brightens your skin. To add a little crunch, you can toss some nuts into soup or sprinkle them over salads.

As far as nuts go, walnuts are the most antioxidant-rich and contain a lot of omega-3 fats. They are a great anti-inflammatory snack for better skin (and overall health) because of this combination.

Additionally beneficial to your digestive system are walnuts. Skin health is directly tied to the health of our microbiota, and excellent gut health helps the skin maintain homeostasis for optimal protection, temperature control, and fluid retention.

4. Chocolates with a dark flavor

Indeed! Favorite chocolates are healthy since they contain even more antioxidants than berries. Consuming chocolate in moderation can have anti-aging benefits. They have powerful antioxidants called cocoa flavanols that shield your skin from the sun. Additionally, it improves skin hydration and nourishes your skin by increasing blood flow, which further protects your skin. Make sure the chocolate you select is just dark and contains at least 70% cocoa.

A great source of magnesium, another anti-inflammatory mineral, is dark chocolate. Magnesium improves the length and quality of sleep, reduces stress, and delays the aging process of the skin. Just be careful to check how much sugar is added to your favorite dark chocolate bar—too much sugar might lead to skin issues.

According to a study from Baylor University College of Medicine, sugar negatively affects collagen fibers and can make the skin appear less elastic and stiff.

5. Carrots

Unbeknownst to many, sweet potatoes are excellent for skin health. Its high vitamin A content helps to repair damaged collagen, preventing wrinkles and fine lines. Consuming foods high in vitamin A, such as sweet potatoes, can also make you seem radiant. Just toss them in the oven for around 35 minutes, spritzing them with extra virgin olive oil, salt, and pepper.

6. Tomatoes

Tomato and tomato juice are high in lycopene, a natural carotenoid that protects skin from sun radiation. Raw tomatoes are not as good as cooked or processed ones.

7: Oily fish

Omega-3 fatty acids are abundant in fatty fish, including salmon, mackerel, and tuna, and are crucial for healthy, radiant skin. These fats are also essential for reducing skin inflammation and moisturizing your skin.

These fish are high in vitamin E and zinc, which have the ability to heal wounds and soothe irritation and acne.

8: **Wine of the red variety**

Fantastic news! Red wine is a tonic that delays aging. It makes you appear younger. Red wine may enhance your heart health, lower your blood pressure, give you radiant skin, and more, according to research. Drinking one or two glasses of red wine every day may have remarkable anti-aging benefits.

Following this healthful guidance results in a better body and mind, in addition to younger-looking skin and greater radiance. In addition, remember that no matter what you eat, getting enough sleep, exercising, and wearing sunscreen are still important.

Foods to restrict your intake of

Deep-fried Food

Diets high in fat and excess fat can cause blood flow problems in the skin, which can lead to wrinkles and early aging. Your liver eliminates toxins from your body naturally when it is working properly.

On the other hand, if these toxins build up in your liver and aren't sufficiently broken down, they might damage your skin, leading to redness, dehydration, puffiness, wrinkles, sallowness, acne, and elasticity loss.

Processed salt

Consuming too much processed salt might hasten the aging process of your skin and body. It is commonly ingested through food items such as cheese, pepperoni, pizza, chips, crackers, cereals, and so on. When taken excessively late at night, it causes the body to retain water and bloat. You'll wake up the next day feeling bloated and dehydrated if your midnight snack was a bag of chips or anything else very salty. This occurs as a result of dehydration brought on by the shrinking of body cells. Dehydration speeds up the aging process and results in wrinkles on the skin.

Meat

A high-protein diet that maintains your health and aids in muscular growth is meat. On the other side, eating processed meats like bacon, sausages, and deli meat might dehydrate you and reduce your body's ability to produce vitamin C, which is needed to make collagen and slow down the aging process.

Things you should be aware of about yourself

1. **Regaining Your Face's Vibrancy by Flattering Your Hair**

Cutting and styling your hair to reduce aging signs is the key to flattering your hair. Maintaining a youthful appearance can be undermined if you keep wearing haircuts that are more appropriate for a younger person. For this reason, as women age, they frequently start to modify their hairdo, usually to something shorter.

These fine lines are usually more noticeable at the upper part of your face, though occasionally they also emerge in the lower area as your skin becomes thinner and wrinkles appear.

There are numerous ways to make your appearance appear years younger with a change in hair color and style. Here are a few instances of how wearing hair that flatters you can make you appear much younger:

2. Make use of the color wheel's power.

Our hair changes color as we get older. Certain alterations are minor, like our hair color becoming lighter with time. While some hair color changes—like graying or even white hair—can be quite noticeable,.

Avoiding using a hair color that makes your hair appear much darker is one way to combat this indication of aging and look younger. A hair color choice that is too dark can draw attention to lines on the face, neck, and forehead, in addition to being easily identified as coloring.

To make your gray hair blend in naturally, go for a lighter color when trying to make your hair look younger. In this setting, the gray hairs provide the impression of highlights, which deepens your color.

It's critical to acknowledge that as you age, you should begin to brighten or enhance your current hair color rather than attempting to stay with the same hue for the majority of your life. By adding brightness and gloss that complement your new skin tone, lightening your hair as you age can help you counteract pigmentation changes in your skin.

By following this easy trick, you can look years younger and feel much more assured about your physical attractiveness as you get older.

3. Change Up Your Look: Draw Attention to and Dress Your Age

You can detract from your obvious aging signs with accessories that go well with a classic, stylish outfit.

Jiggling upper arms can be disguised with a chic sweater, while drooping neck skin can be covered up with a simple silk scarf that goes well with your outfit.

You might deflect attention by wearing eye-catching jewelry or brilliant pendants on your breastplate. However, make sure that the necklaces you wear to appear younger are not too tight; as you age, necklaces should be longer, hanging just above the breast but as far below the face as possible.

Make sure you wear age-appropriate attire while choosing outfits that will make you appear younger.

When you get older, the slimming dress that you were able to fit into as a young lady could lose its attractiveness. When you dress too young for your body type, you may actually look older than you actually are by exposing portions of your body that naturally age.

4. **Discover these tricks for having eyes that look younger.**

Are there any particular signs of aging on your face that are causing you significant discomfort? You're not alone; we all are. However, there are a few simple tricks you may do to hide the aging signs and appear younger:

1. **a) Subtle Cosmetics Can Hide Crow's Feet**

The infamous lines that develop next to our eyes as we age are called "crow's feet." This is a confidence-killer for a lot of women, who would rather hide it to appear younger and feel more assured.

Proper use of cosmetics can help you conceal the following facial aging signs:

Crow's feet

Creases

Underneath, eye pigmentation

Deep creases

Even though you can't totally hide wrinkles with makeup, you can make them less noticeable by dabbing concealer around your eyes only where it's needed. Caution: Excessive use of powder or foundation on the crow's feet may actually make them more noticeable.

1. b) Be aware of the appropriate dark eye circle treatments.

Applying concealer to the region around your eyes that has discoloration, such as dark circles, can be facilitated by using a small, flat makeup brush. In an attempt to mix the concealer, you risk straining the skin around your eyes by massaging it in, which will exacerbate some signs of aging.

Collagen depletion over time is the cause of the excess skin and discoloration under the eyes. This is the stuff that gives you tight, firm skin. You can also think about using some natural cures to increase the amount of collagen in your diet, which will make you seem at least ten years younger.

1. c) Get Rid of Droopy Eyes

Your eyelids begin to sag as they become heavier over time. This may result in bags under your eyes, making them appear smaller. The volume and color of our eyebrows and eyelashes gradually fade with age, which lessens the contrast required to make you appear awake. An extremely thick coat of mascara will draw attention away from your lash line and elongate your eye.

In old age, some people may start to feel sagging of the forehead and upper eyelids. In fact, this may result in visual issues and make you appear much older. Botox and liquid facelifts are great ways to help you seem years younger by reducing these indications of aging.

5. Take Care of Your Skin: Throughout Your Life, It Makes a Big Difference

As we age, we must take better care of our skin by adhering to a regular cleansing and exfoliating routine. By doing this, you'll help eliminate extra layers of dead skin cells from your face as well as stimulate the production of more collagen and antioxidants to support the creation of new cells.

This is a natural technique to naturally enhance shine and vibrancy in your appearance, as it will consistently reveal the brighter skin cells underlying it. You may reduce the look of your face by at least ten years by using these easy tricks for looking younger.

Maintaining hydration will also help you get greater outcomes because it will allow your body to actively remove toxins and provide your skin with more nutrients. Because exercise increases blood flow and causes perspiration to clear the pores, it has also been demonstrated to help lessen the appearance of aging skin on the face.

Finally, there are a few more simple tactics and advice for looking younger that you may apply on a regular basis to keep your face looking young:

Every day, moisturize.

When required, wear sunscreen.

Consume meals that improve the health of your skin.

We'll go into more detail about a few meals that can make you feel and look younger later in this book.

You are, after all, what you eat!

6. Avoid Toxins in Your Environment and Diet

Eliminating any preventable toxins from your environment and diet should be a part of your skin care regimen. It goes without saying that some things are just inescapable. As an illustration, let's say you work in a job that exposes you to high amounts of air pollution or you live in an urban location.

But even under these kinds of circumstances, you can look younger by ridding your body and skin of these undesirable, toxic substances.

It is essential that you stay out of the sun as much as possible, regardless of the weather. You can include sun protection accessories, such as hats, into your outfit to keep it stylish and timeless. Additionally, you ought to wear sunscreen on your face at all times, or at the very least, use lotions or makeup that offer UV protection.

Because toxins can affect you from all directions, not just

the sun, it's critical to stay away from activities like smoking and being near secondhand smoke. The majority of the over 4,000 known carcinogens and compounds found in cigarette smoke attach themselves to water molecules, which makes your skin an ideal place for them to wreak havoc.

Aging can be accelerated by driving in heavy traffic, leaving your windows down, and taking other unnecessary risks that expose you to pollutants in the environment. If your line of work or environment requires it, make sure to exfoliate your skin on a regular basis to help rid your skin of these toxic pollutants.

Our meals also contain contaminants that may have an impact on how we age. You must make an effort to stay away from the following meals and beverages if you want to appear ten years younger:

booze

Candies

Trans Fats

Coffee

You'll increase your chances of aging more gradually by taking these easy steps to look and feel younger while lowering your exposure to pollutants.

7. Certain drugs can make you appear younger.

Consider upgrading your skin care routine if you truly want to appear years younger. Skin care products with prescription strength can help restore and nourish your skin. Recall that every modern medication we use for medical conditions contains a natural or plant-based derivative. Mother Nature can assist you in the form of a powerful prescription, so don't be afraid of her.

For instance, retinoid is essentially a form of vitamin A that occurs naturally in dairy products, eggs, and meat. Any creams or face care products that contain this derivative will help shield your skin from the effects of aging. It is a vitamin that is vital for the health of your skin.

Age spots, sun spots, and other symptoms of aging can be reversed with the use of pigment controls.

When natural means of hydrating the skin prove insufficient, a hydrator can aid.

Supplementing with antioxidants can enhance the nutritional value of the foods you eat, and using sunscreen can shield you from sun damage while still supplying your body with the appropriate amount of vitamin D.

8. Attempts Completed, But Nothing Happens? Non-surgical methods may be beneficial.

Everyone has the right to feel and look their best. If you've tried every trick in the book to seem younger and nothing has worked, there are a few extremely reasonably priced non-surgical cosmetic procedures that can help you regain your confidence.

1. a) Allow skin-brightening procedures to make your life happier.

With just a few procedures, skin-brightening techniques including microdermabrasion, light peels, micro laser peels, and the Clear & Brilliant laser treatment can make patients appear at least ten years younger.

The following therapies can be applied to counteract facial aging signs:

creases

Age-related spots

Lines

1. b) Restore skin that's old and sunburned.

Chemical peels or laser skin resurfacing are two methods for treating sun-damaged skin. These treatments can be used to repair medium-to-deep wrinkles, eliminate discoloration, and restore pigmentation to parts of the skin affected by the sun, depending on your situation.

These non-surgical procedures, which take about an hour to complete, are quick, simple, almost painless, and help patients look younger than their actual age.

1. c) Replumb lost facial fullness

As we age, our faces lose volume, which can lead to skin sagging and hollowness in certain areas, particularly around the cheekbones. In order to counteract this, dermal fillers, injectable fillers, and even fat transfers can be used to increase volume beneath the outermost layers of skin, where collagen is no longer present.

In order to ensure optimal outcomes and correct execution, all of these operations ought to be carried out by a highly skilled specialist. For individuals who wish to look younger without having surgery, these therapies are perfect.

1. d) Tighten and lift loose facial skin.

Sagging facial skin can be lifted and tightened using non-surgical or surgical methods. One non-surgical method is a liquid facelift, in which the lost volume is naturally made up for by injecting liquid into the face by a master injector.

The effects of these anti-aging procedures start to diminish after only around a year. However, those who wish to test cosmetic treatments for the first time frequently choose them over surgical facelifts.

Surgical techniques such as facelifts, necklifts, eyelid surgeries, and brow lifts remove extra skin, minimize wrinkles indirectly, and tighten the skin to make aging symptoms less noticeable.

1. How to Appear Ten Years Younger in Your Body

Although the face is the main place where people see the effects of aging, our bodies also have a significant impact on how old we appear and how other people see us. In this section, I will describe several useful strategies and tricks you may apply to make your body look a decade younger.

9. Increase Your Movement: Exercise Is Essential for a Healthy Body

It has been demonstrated that regular exercise and easy stretches can reduce the physical indicators of aging. Here are some simple techniques you may use to keep your body looking younger and boost your confidence:

Getting 20 minutes of exercise every day

Moving more often

Rather than sitting at your desk, stand up.

taking a stroll outside

ensuring that you walk 10,000 steps or more each day.

These easy techniques will all significantly improve your circulation and blood flow. Your body as a whole receives more nutrients from this, which aids in:

Preserve the diminishing muscle mass that ages you.

Luminize the skin.

Sweating can aid in the removal of toxins.

And a lot more...

Being active and exercising makes you feel younger in addition to making you look younger. Keeping up a consistent fitness routine is crucial to feeling more confident, energetic, and at ease with our bodies as we age.

10.   Keep Up a Healthy Diet: Your Food Reflects Who You Are!

The proverb "you are what you eat" is well known to all of us. To tell the truth, this proverb is often accurate. If you regularly consume foods high in:

Sugars

processed sugars

Trans fats

and other extras.

You will probably be in worse shape than someone who eats a well-balanced meal.

This poor diet will therefore also affect how old you seem as you get older. People who maintain unhealthy diets and exercise routines throughout their 20s, 30s, and 40s are unlikely to age as gracefully as those who do not.

So what are the vitamins and nutrients that your body certainly requires to maintain a youthful appearance in old age? What food should you eat to feel and look ten years younger?

All diets designed to make you look younger center on four essential vitamins:

Vitamin A

Vitamin C

D-vitamine

Vitamin E

Let's examine these vitamins in more detail to learn how they keep you looking young and what foods you should be consuming to do the same.

11.   Remember that over 70% of our bodies are made of water.

Staying well hydrated throughout the day will increase your physical performance, lower your maximum heart rate, and lessen weariness.

Furthermore, hydration elevates your mood by lowering feelings of exhaustion, disorientation, and drowsiness. You might feel calmer and more positive by lowering your bad feelings. One of the main causes of the appearance of aging is stress, which has been linked to:

Graying hair

Hair thinning

Wrinkles and lines on the forehead

A rise in cardiovascular issues

Plus additional...

Naturally, you won't be able to achieve the youthful appearance you desire if you are always stressed out. Furthermore, long-term stress can lead to hormone imbalances, which can exacerbate the indications of aging.

Additional research suggests that staying hydrated enhances cognitive function.

Regardless of age, drinking more water will enhance performance when performing cognitive tasks.

Finally, maintaining hydration aids in the delivery of water to all of your cells, including those in your skin. Water is one of the best methods to seem younger since it helps you maintain your skin's volume, brightness, and healing over time. These benefits can pile up over time.

12.   Take in a good amount of sunlight, but be careful of burns.

Because the sun produces vitamin D, it helps maintain healthy bones, skin, and hair. This vital anti-aging vitamin aids in the body's absorption of calcium, which is required for healthy bone formation.

Osteoporosis is a major worry for the elderly, particularly women. Using an appropriate sunscreen, 30 minutes of daily sun exposure can help to improve bone density and fight the symptoms of aging.

The best thing about this method for seeming ten years younger is that it costs nothing at all. All you need to do is head outdoors to take a tranquil siesta under the sun.

13.   Get More Sleep: 7- to 8-hour sleep is typical.

Sleep helps to maintain general cognitive function and physical wellness. It promotes growth in all age groups, and getting enough sleep helps you feel better emotionally and have more energy during the day. Consequently, you will be able to:

Increase your level of activity and exercise.

Lower your stress levels.

Reduce the aging symptoms.

Generally, in order to maintain normal physical processes, most doctors advise people to receive between 7 and 8 hours of sleep per night. This implies that you are essentially losing out on your beauty sleep if you typically get less sleep than this!

This is just another easy tip you may use to look young as you get older.

14.   Maintain Hormone Balance: As We Age, Our Hormones Change

Our bodies no longer replace some hormones as effectively as they previously did as we age.

We start this process when we turn thirty, and it lasts the remainder of our lives.

This is something that many women go through later in life, during the menopause, when their bodies start to change and they produce far less estrogen. This shift in hormone production can significantly affect how old a person feels and looks. Furthermore, for some women, this might cause excruciating discomfort throughout menopause.

This shift in hormone levels in males may cause them to feel lethargic and have trouble achieving sexual pleasure. A harder time gaining and maintaining muscular mass may also follow as testosterone levels continue to drop.

It has been demonstrated that there is a way for both men and women to regain some of their youthful appearance, energy, and confidence as they age. One treatment that a licensed cosmetic surgeon can provide is hormone replacement therapy (HRT). The goal of this treatment is to restore confidence in older men and women.

1. The Mind: How to Feel Younger as You Age

I was compelled to add this section because I believe that

many of us become so preoccupied with fighting and worrying about the outward manifestations of aging as we age that we neglect to consider one of the most significant aspects of aging—our minds.

The following advice will make you feel younger even as you age, which will have a positive impact on how you look and how you interact with others on a regular basis. I think that maintaining a youthful mindset as we age is just as vital as continuing to eat well and exercise.

15.   Reduce Your Stress: It's Not Worth It

Just as stress eats away at our bodies, it also eats away at our minds. Thus, try not to overstress yourself. Your brain will eventually shrink due to the death of brain cells brought on by excessive stress. Reduce your stress levels since long-term stress shrinks your prefrontal cortex, the area of the brain required for memory and/or learning.

Several easy actions you may take every day to lower your stress levels include:

Steer clear of excessive caffeine use.

Inhale deeply.

Engage in regular exercise.

Continue eating healthfully.

Recall your blessings.

Take a rest.

In other words, tension is not worth it. It will probably take up other aspects of your life and make you feel and appear older than you actually are. Breathe deeply, acknowledge your blessings, and take a moment to yourself if necessary.

16.   Try New Things: Avoid Being Stuck

When people stop being physically, spiritually, and cognitively active, some indicators of aging can occur very quickly. Even though these are all very significant issues, we frequently mistake the quick deterioration of our bodies and minds for age-related issues.

You push the brain to clear the plaque from between the neurons in your neural connections as you keep learning new things. This keeps your mind as clear-cut as it was in your younger years.

Like all the other muscles in the body, neurons can expand and contract.

However, if you don't exercise them, they won't do that. It's natural to feel uncomfortable while trying something new, but if you push past that initial feeling of unease or fear, you will:

Develop new neuronal growth.

Take out the plaque.

Take precautions to avoid conditions like Alzheimer's.

And help fuel your thoughts.

You don't have to quit doing things because you're getting older. To maintain your youthful appearance and mental acuity, do something new once a week or once a month.

17.   Be certain: Respecting one's age is important. It's critical to embrace your age and have self-assurance. Nothing will totally stop the aging process, but if you are successful in appearing younger, you should be happy with it. Your confidence will radiate from the inside out, the more you believe in yourself and your accomplishments. Beauty transcends the surface.

I occasionally advise people who are having confidence issues to try something else.

Consider taking a trip, doing something different, or simply getting a new haircut.

At other times, your companion is a source of confidence. Maybe tell them how you're feeling and ask for their validation regarding your appearance.

It might be time to think about getting some anti-aging cosmetic procedures done if you are having trouble regaining your confidence and are really self-conscious about the way your body is changing. Everyone has the right to embrace their body and feel confident in it. It's important to consult a specialist to figure out how to appear and feel younger if you feel like you've tried everything and nothing is working.

Thinking of having cosmetic surgery to appear younger?

We are all ultimately growing older every second. This usually translates into looking older as well. Even though aging is an inevitable process, there are still things you can do to control how you appear.

We covered a variety of non-surgical and surgical cosmetic procedures in this post that can make you appear ten years younger. Take our cosmetic self-evaluation below to find out more about these procedures and how they can give you a younger-looking appearance.

This brief assessment will assist you in learning more about:

Which process works best for you?

What actions should I take next?

Or, get in touch with us right now to schedule a consultation with me, Dr. Larry Fan, if you'd like to talk to a specialist about customized procedures that can make you feel and look younger. As a board-certified plastic surgeon, I have helped men and women from all over the nation feel more confident about their appearance by doing over 5,000 cosmetic procedures on them. Additionally, for ten years running, I have been selected as one of America's top plastic surgeons.

I'm sure I have the knowledge and expertise to help you solve any issue you're having and look younger than you are right now.

Section Seven

Advantages of growing older

As we age, we have access to a greater feeling of acceptance of ourselves and others, the means to form the connection we desire, life experiences that guide our decisions, knowledge, and empathy. Remember to be grateful as well.

Many of the symptoms we associate with aging, such as pain and memory loss, are difficult to accept and have come to represent stereotypes associated with aging. But since we're living longer and frequently in better condition, we realize that we get better with age in a lot of aspects.

As we age, we have access to a greater feeling of acceptance of ourselves and others, the means to form the connection we desire, life experiences that guide our decisions, knowledge, and empathy.

Remember to be grateful as well. As we age, we can become more appreciative of our family and our financial, emotional, and physical well-being, which helps us to just be happy to be alive.

Physiological age versus chronological age

Davangere P. Devanand, MD, teaches neurology and psychiatry at Columbia University's Vagelos College of Physicians and Surgeons and serves as the director of geriatric psychiatry. He emphasizes that age is merely a number, even if it is our chronological age. What truly distinguishes people as middle-aged or older is their physiological age, such as cardiac function, for example.

According to biological indicators, Devanand notes, "some people in their 30s to 50s may have poor health for various reasons, and they are old." "Those who are the same age chronologically do not age in the same way; instead, they maintain excellent health and fitness."

Improvements when one ages

The survival effect may account for some of the advantages of aging that we associate with it. According to Devanand,

"Those who get older are the survivors and are more resilient." Others may pass away due to illnesses, mishaps, suicide, drug misuse, or other uncontrollable circumstances. Those elder survivors are less likely to be sad or have substance addiction problems than many of their younger peers.

Nevertheless, our minds might become sharper as we get older. According to Devanand, "the traditional IQ test is used to measure raw intelligence, and older people may have a slight decline because of memory loss." "As we age, we lose certain connections—how we remember and put things in context."

It is nevertheless feasible to acquire new knowledge. It is a common occurrence when elderly individuals pick up new technology, including laptops and smartphones. Younger individuals, he says, "seem to have more space on their mental hard drives," so it just appears easier to them.

According to him, social and emotional intelligence do tend to get better with age. "Those who are older tend to be less volatile emotionally, have a deeper comprehension of

relationships, and have developed coping mechanisms for various circumstances—a quality known as wisdom."

For humans to be able to survive, their fight-or-flight response depends on specific brain nerve cells. However, as we get older, the quantity of these cells in the brain's locus ceruleus and sympathetic nervous system may fall to half, which reduces our capacity to produce anxiety. For instance, panic attacks are common in younger people, but because those neurons just disappear beyond the age of 60 or 65, new-onset panic disorder is uncommon and practically unheard of, according to Devanand.

As we age, our response times generally increase, which can be problematic in scenarios like traffic. A longer response time, however, allows an older person more time to examine the issue and provide a well-thought-out solution. "Having more time reduces impulsivity, which can be a major issue for a lot of younger people," he claims. Understanding the causes and effects of many circumstances comes from experience in life.

"And as we age, we become more skilled at managing a range of issues, which may also enable greater tolerance in general."

As people age, they have more opportunities for social connection and community involvement since they can live in retirement communities with infinite social events or use senior facilities. "Older people prefer to have a larger circle and view social relationships from a broad perspective," he explains. Many of those older, more reclusive people managed to maintain their optimistic view during the pandemic by using Zoom and other virtual tools. "They know that having a narrow circle may make them more depressed." "They managed to maintain their resilience and stay connected."

Is this an illness or just normal aging?

According to Devanand, if progress in public health and medicine continues, the average human may live to be over 100 years old. He states, "It may be hard to imagine now, but it's theoretically possible."

It's frequently challenging to distinguish between illness and normal aging.

For instance, nearly everyone experiences an increase in blood pressure with age; is this a sign of sickness or normal aging? This also applies to memory loss. Most people struggle to recall names, locations, and other details, but is this typical or indicative of Alzheimer's disease?

"The majority of people would have high blood pressure and many would have Alzheimer's disease if the average person lived to be 100 years of age or more, but that's an ongoing medical debate," he says. "One's functional impairment would just bc different in severity."

Devanand continues, "It will take work in one's younger years to maintain quality of life as one ages." It is well established that maintaining cognitive function and lowering the risk of heart disease and stroke can be achieved with regular exercise and a balanced diet. Additionally, social interactions are critical to both mental and physical health.

"Health is not a given; how we age is determined by the amount of work we put into our food and exercise routines.

Physical well-being frequently necessitates taking extra precautions.

The Top 10 Benefits of Getting Older

Like any stage of life, being a senior can have obstacles. But all the good things about becoming older shouldn't be overshadowed by the challenging and unpleasant aspects of aging.

The Greatest Things About Getting Older

Here is a list of ten wonderful things about getting older, ranging from the financial benefits of reaching 65 to the life lessons gained from decades of experience:

1. A more optimistic outlook

Studies reveal that seniors are among the happiest age groups, with a much higher level of happiness than those in their middle years, which may surprise some.

Dr. Saverio Stranges, the author of a study on the topic, speculates that this might be because of improved coping mechanisms. Seniors may also be happier because they are "more comfortable being themselves" as they get older, which is another reason why older individuals typically have internal systems to deal with hardship or unfavorable conditions better than younger ones.

2. Grandkids

As American writer Gore Vidal once quipped, "Never have children, only grandchildren." Often, grandparents get to enjoy all the good things about having little children without having to deal with night terrors and changing diapers. Grandparents adore their grandkids, and this love helps the grandchildren who receive it as well as lightening the grandparents' own hearts.

Dr. Karl Pillemer, who specializes in the study of aging and the relationships between generations, firmly believes that the bond between a kid and their grandparents is important. He states that the grandparent-grandchild relationship is the second most important relationship in terms of emotional significance, after the parent-child relationship, and that "research shows children need four to six involved, caring adults in their lives to fully develop emotionally and socially."

3. Extended time with loved ones

Retirement isn't automatically happy or soothing; what makes it unique is how you spend your time there.

Spending time with loved ones, friends, and family during retirement is one of the nicest aspects of the lifestyle.

4. Possibility of Following Your Dreams

Retirement is a great chance to rekindle passions and goals that you may have put on hold. Victorian novelist George Elliot once said, "It's never too late to be what you might have become."

For example, you may create the novel that has been sitting in your head waiting to be released, travel to a place you've always wanted to visit, or pick up a new language.

5. Civic Engagement and Volunteering

Being older gives one a wider perspective, and it frequently encourages people to devote a large portion of their time and resources to improving society and the environment for coming generations.

Retired seniors have more time to engage in politics and the community, which they do in addition to spending time

with loved ones and pursuing hobbies and personal goals. For example, adults over the age of 65 vote at a higher rate than any other age group, according to data from the U.S. Bureau of Census. Additionally, they volunteer a lot. According to data from the Bureau of Labor and Statistics, one in four American seniors 65 and older engaged in volunteer work in 2015.

6. Knowledge

Many recent studies illustrating the cognitive and emotional advantages of aging were highlighted in an article published in Smithsonian Magazine. Seniors are more adept at managing their emotions than people in other age groups, according to a study mentioned in the article. A gambling game "designed to induce regret" was administered to participants of all ages by the researchers, who discovered that "those in their 60s didn't agonize over losing, and they were less likely to try to redeem their loss by later taking big risks," in contrast to 20-somethings.

Visit our blog post "Priceless Advice from Older Americans" to read some excellent counsel from the most knowledgeable people in America.

7. Enhancing social skills and increasing empathy

In a different study referenced in the previously mentioned article, participants were asked to advise made-up writers of "Dear Abby" letters. The results showed that elders have better social and empathy skills. According to the study:

"Those in their 60s demonstrated superior ability to envision divergent viewpoints, consider various solutions, and make concession suggestions compared to younger participants."

Elderly people are susceptible to isolation, even though they may have developed stronger social skills than their younger counterparts. To ensure that these abilities have an opportunity to flourish, read our blog post about assisting elders in avoiding social isolation.

8. Guaranteed Minimum Wage, Social Security, and Medicare

In a piece on the history of aging, we talked about how, prior to the turn of the 20th century, elderly people who were unable to support themselves were compelled to live in what were known as "workhouses" or "poorhouses."

These individuals were either dependent on their families for care or were not independently wealthy.

Even though senior poverty is still a major issue, safety net programs like Medicare, Medicaid, and Social Security ensure that all American seniors, regardless of their financial situation or lack of dependent children, have access to health insurance and a guaranteed minimum income.

In 1935, President Franklin D. Roosevelt stated, "We can never insure one-hundred percent of the population against one-hundred percent of the hazards and vicissitudes of life," in describing the significance of Social Security and other safety-net programs that he assisted in enacting. However, we have made an effort to draft legislation that will provide some level of protection to the typical citizen and his family against job loss and old-age poverty.

9. Senior Savings

Even though senior discounts seem insignificant, you must have once envied them. Senior discounts can help people save money during a time when income is often fixed and restricted.

Because the discounts are frequently applied to the exact services—such as dining, medicine, entertainment, and transportation—that support seniors in maintaining an active and involved lifestyle, they also serve as a fantastic motivator for seniors to make the most of their retirement. Seniors can even find companies that provide senior discounts by using websites such as SeniorDiscounts.com.

10. Feeling of Achievement

An appropriately healthy sense of pride in their accomplishments is common among older adults. These achievements don't have to be enormous.

John Lennon's lyric, "A working-class hero is something to be," explains it perfectly. Apparently commonplace accomplishments, such as having a healthy and happy kid, being happily married, defending the country, or leaving a position with good standing after years of hard work, can serve as the cornerstone for a joyful and contented old age.

Synopsis: Transformation, Rejuvenation, and Aging

1. Amphibian metamorphosis encompasses modifications in both morphology and biochemistry. A new structure is created, some are replaced, and some are modified.

2. During amphibian metamorphosis, many changes are unique to a given area. The head epidermis remains intact, while the tail epidermis dies. An eye can be transplanted into a dying tail and yet survive.

3. Thyroxine (T4) and triiodothyronine (T3), two thyroid hormones, are the ones that cause amphibian metamorphosis. Early alterations that take place at low thyroid hormone concentrations seem to be the cause of the coordination of metamorphic changes. We refer to this as the threshold idea. The potential of thyroid hormones to stimulate the synthesis of more thyroid hormone receptor proteins may serve as the biological underpinning for the autoinduction of thyroid hormones. The primary mode of action of thyroid hormones is transcriptional.

4. Changing the relative pace of growth in various animal parts is known as heterochrony. The tadpole stage is no longer present in animals that have direct development. For example, certain frogs develop limbs while still in the egg.

5. Neoteny is characterized by a slowing of the juvenile (larval) form while the gonads and germ cells mature normally. During progenesis, the body's other tissues mature normally, but the gonads and germ cells mature quickly. The animal can mate in both situations when it is still a larva.

6. In insects that are ametabolous, development occurs directly. In the nymph stage of hemimetabolous insects, the young organism is typically a scaled-down counterpart of the adult. Holometabolous insects undergo a remarkable transformation from larva to pupa to adult sexual maturity.

7. An instar is the stage of a larva that occurs between molts. The larva goes through a metamorphic molt to become a pupa, following the last instar stage. To become an adult, the pupa must go through an instar molt.

8. The imaginal discs and histoblasts develop and differentiate to create the adult body's structures during the pupal stage.

9. The proximal-distal, dorsal-ventral, and anterior-posterior axes are successively determined and entail interactions across several imaginal disc compartments.

10. Hydroxyecdysone is the hormone that causes molting. The molt is an instar molt when there are large amounts of juvenile hormone present. When juvenile hormone levels are low, the molt results in the development of a pupa; when juvenile hormone levels are absent, the molt is known as an imaginary molt.

11. At least three distinct proteins can be formed from nRNA produced by the ecdysone receptor gene. The way a cell reacts to hydroxyecdysone can be influenced by the types of ecdysone receptors present in that cell. To either activate or repress transcription, the ecdysone receptors attach to DNA.

12. Three main categories of regeneration exist. Tissues dedifferentiate into a blastema during epimorphosis (such as the regeneration of limbs), divide, and then redifferentiate into the new form. In morphallaxis, which is a hydra characteristic, there is little to no growth and only a repatterning of the existing tissue. Cells divide during compensatory regeneration while maintaining their differentiated condition, as seen in the liver.

13. An apical ectodermal cap is formed by the epidermis in the regenerated salamander limb. A blastema is formed when the cells underneath it dedifferentiate. The differentiated cells return to the cell cycle after losing their adhesions. Mammals do not experience this.

14. There seem to be gradients related to head activation, head inhibition, foot activity, and foot inhibition in hydras. Where these gradients are the lowest, hydra budding takes place.

15. Researchers studying medicine are examining if paracrine substances allow for local regeneration in mammals. In an attempt to encourage regeneration, embryonic conditions are being restored for bone and brain cells.

16. Recently, natural inhibitors of neural regeneration have been identified; it may be possible to circumvent these inhibitors to allow for spinal cord regeneration.

17. A species' maximum life span is determined by the length of time its oldest known member has lived. It is mostly unique to a certain species. The amount of time that about 50% of a species' individuals live in a particular population is known as life expectancy.

18. We may investigate aging on a number of levels, including genetic, biochemical, and cellular levels. Reactive oxygen species (ROS) have the ability to alter DNA, damage cell membranes, and inactivate proteins. The life span of the mutants can be altered by mutations that affect their capacity to produce or break down ROS.

19. Proteins that control aging may target mitochondria.

20. The decline of physiological capabilities required for survival and reproduction over time is known as aging. It is important to distinguish between senescence-related disorders like cancer and heart disease, which impact individuals, and the phenotypic changes associated with senescence, which affect all members of the species.

www.ingramcontent.com/pod-product-compliance
Lightning Source LLC
Chambersburg PA
CBHW070832250726

48662CB00003B/1188